Medical Journalism

The writer's guide

Medical Journalism

The writer's guide

TIM ALBERT

Consultant and Trainer in Written Communication ; Visiting Lecturer in Medical Journalism, City University, London ; formerly Editor of BMA News Review.

WITH A FOREWORD BY
MICHAEL O'DONNELL

RADCLIFFE MEDICAL PRESS
OXFORD

British Library Cataloguing in Publication Data

Albert, Tim
    Medical Journalism: Writer's Guide
    I. Title
    070.4

    ISBN   1-870905-28-8

Typeset by Bookman, Bristol
Printed and bound in Great Britain by
Biddles Ltd, Guildford and King's Lynn

For Brian Fogg and Mike Tillson, who set me out on this world of journalism, and for Barbara, who has sustained me along the way.

Contents

Foreword

Tim Albert is ideally qualified to write this book. Not only is he an accomplished writer but he's one of the few journalists I know who is also a talented teacher.

My only grouse about the book is that it didn't exist when I first hung up my stethoscope and tried to turn myself into a writer. It would have spared me months of struggle in an alien world where experience eventually taught me some of the lessons I could have learned less traumatically from these pages.

Tim Albert offers straightforward descriptions of the techniques that underpin our craft. But I should warn ingenuous readers that, though the techniques are easy to understand, the problems – and the hard work – come when we try to apply them.

Nearly every cliché uttered about writing is true. (Struggle as we must to keep clichés out of our prose, we can't keep them out of our lives.) So I don't apologize for repeating the truism that the only way to learn how to write is to write, and to keep on writing.

Then, if you have any feeling for words, and can learn to write simply, directly, and with enthusiasm, you are well on the way to the first reward – getting something published.

You'll also discover that, though you understand the need to write simple, direct prose, the need is not easily fulfilled. As one doctor-writer, William Somerset Maugham, put it: 'To write simply is as difficult as to be good.' If anything, he understated the problem.

Yet achieving an appearance of simplicity is the central skill of our craft and experience has taught me that the only way to fashion simple readable prose is to rewrite, rewrite, and rewrite. And then rewrite.

Once you've enjoyed the excitement of getting into print, you may be tempted to make writing your main occupation rather than a part-time one. If so, be warned that once you start writing for a living, you can't rely only on technique.

You'll need to cultivate a way of living that feeds your imagination.

And you'll need to indulge in some cold-blooded introspection to try to discover more about the creature who produces the words, the voice that speaks to the reader when you write. For, unless you write with some honesty of purpose, and try honestly to express the complexities within you and which you see around you, your writing will smack of triteness. To write from any motive other than honesty is to write propaganda. That may not deter you because propaganda is a profitable form of writing. It demands the same skills and techniques as any other writing and those who produce it are well paid. Some professionals produce it to buy time to write what they really want to write and it does them little harm as long as they retain insight into what they're doing and why.

Sometimes, however, beguiled by good pay and work that's not too demanding, they do lose insight. And that's a pity. For propaganda is thin gruel to sustain the enthusiasm of a full-time writer. And you can measure its charm by reading advertising brochures or watching party political broadcasts.

The only drawback to being a professional writer is actually having to write. I've yet to meet anyone who finds the business of setting down words a pleasurable way of passing the time and all of us yearn for some diversion that will take us away from the desk or keyboard – or better still, will prevent us from even starting.

Our craft, I'm sad to report, demands self-discipline and most writers I know compel themselves to write a certain number of words – or to spend a specified time at their desk – every day. Some of the best prose they produce may come during a session that got off to a reluctant start while some sessions that grew out of bubbling enthusiasm may produce only rubbish.

Because the execution can be such a chore, writers of all sorts, but particularly journalists, need occasional assurance that they aren't mere reporters of other people's activities but serve some useful purpose of their own.

I happen to believe that they do because, the longer I live, the more convinced I grow that the only safe place for authority in a free society is on the defensive. And one of a writer's jobs is to keep it there.

It's certainly why we need good medical writers. Doctors are so inept at coping with authority that power within our profession is exerted largely through a mixture of patronage and politesse. If you want an example of the undue deference to which we've been conditioned, listen the next time a visiting notable is introduced at a medical meeting. The language used would seem extravagant in an obituary.

Repeated doses of that sort of stuff tend to encourage pomposity amongst our senior citizens. And once pomposity takes root, the prognosis is pretty grim. That's why we need writers who, when they listen to doctors, can help their readers distinguish between platitudes and wisdom.

We also need writers who can keep a sharp edge on our profession's scepticism. Doctors claim to be scientists, if not exclusively at least in part. Yet, maybe because we've built such impressive monuments to science, with marble pillars at the entrance and laurel-wreathed busts in the hall, we're inclined to forget that science is a subversive trade. Its practitioners expand our knowledge by questioning our certainties and it's up to writers to encourage them in their subversion. At a time when many of the world's troubles are caused by people who have the courage of their convictions, it may be no bad thing to encourage more people to have the courage of their doubts.

One last admonition. If, once you know about the techniques, your enthusiasm – or do I mean obsession? – remains undiminished, then sit down and write ... and keep on writing. Don't talk about it. Don't theorize about it. Just do it. The only acceptable definition of a writer is someone who writes.

MICHAEL O'DONNELL

Preface

Over the past few years, I have spent more and more time talking to doctors who wanted to know about journalism. It really started when I was at *BMA News Review*, when Dr Lyndy Matthews, then a senior house officer, came to spend several months working with us. It continued with a successful series of weekends on medical journalism sponsored by (as they were then) Smith Kline and French. It has now become one of the main parts of my working life, with formal courses and a constant stream of informal queries.

This book was conceived as an attempt to bring together enough information to allow doctors, or other health workers, to start exploring this world of medical journalism. It includes much of the basic information given to any new journalist, but, I hope, adapted to the particular needs and values of the medical professions. I have not missed the irony that their growing interest in medical journalism has coincided with increased complaints that they have forgotten the art of clear medical communication. Without wishing to enter this debate on such an early page, I am conscious that the message in this book has a wider application.

I must thank all those doctors, too many to name, whose interest and shared enthusiasm have stimulated me over these years. I would also like to thank all those, from literary agents to librarians, who have helped me formulate the answers to their many queries. I am particularly grateful to those who have read this book in one form or another, and who have encouraged me to continue: Dr Michael O'Donnell, Dr Gordon Macpherson, Liz McCallum, Dot Peskin, Dr Harvey Marcovitch, Mark Jessop, Helen Parker, Tony Thistlethwaite and Dr Cyril Haxton. As the formula goes, however, all errors are mine.

Finally I would like to thank Andrew Bax and his staff for their help and support, and in particular for believing me when I suggested that this book would meet a need.

TIM ALBERT
February 1992

1   The World of Writing

'Don't believe people who tell you that writing is easy', **Alex Paton**[1].

The aim of this book is to get you writing and published. If you have not written already, use it as a starter kit, to find out what demands this crazy ambition will make, what rewards it will give, and how you can proceed along the path of getting your kicks from seeing your name in print. If you are one of those whose by-line already appears as regularly as long words in a management memo, don't stop reading. This book is intended to reinforce your addiction, clarify your thoughts – if only through disagreeing with some of mine – and improve some of your skills. If there are any writers who insist that their work can never be improved, I would say to them, now is the time to give up and perfect something else.

This book does not offer a magic formula for making the writing process easier: I am afraid that I take the Calvinistic view that the value of an activity increases in proportion to the anguish that goes into it. However, it should give you a better chance of reaching that delightful state of 'having written', which, after food and sex, appears to be one of life's greater satisfactions.

Some argue that good writers are born and not made, and that writing skills cannot be taught. I disagree. There is an element of talent, and some have a greater capacity than others to analyze situations, order thoughts, and use telling words and phrases. Such people can still be encouraged to do things better, while those apparently 'less talented' can be shown how to find marketable ideas, discipline their thoughts, develop an effective writing style and deal competently with editors. It is largely a question of attitude and confidence: '...very few people are incurably bad writers by nature, just as very few are congenitally diseased or deformed'[2]. In the unlikely event that you never get published – though I should make it clear that there is no money-back guarantee with this book – you should find that your writing will have improved, and that you are communicating more effectively with patients and colleagues. You may not be famous, but you should have more time and less aggravation.

All professionals – and health professionals are no exception – tend to write in their own private language. This excerpt from a medical journal gives the flavour:

> 'Therapists rely heavily upon intuition, in the absence of any theory with sufficient explanatory power, to identify and follow recurring sequences of interpersonal behaviour which are seen when family members interact and to understand and predict how and when change in beliefs and behaviour may come about. An intuitive understanding of how to keep in communication with each member of the family is guided by a personally selected blend of congenial concepts which predict how change will come about.'

Cynics will argue that professionals encourage this private language because it promotes their own importance. (Has anyone else noticed the positive correlation between the length of words in a legal document and the level of fee?) With doctors, however, there is a more prosaic reason: from the age of 16 they are taught in the language of science. This puts the blame neatly on the education system.

Here I must distinguish between technical/ scientific language, which has its uses, and jargon, which has none. Often this is a question not of which words you choose, but of which audience you are addressing. The term 'myocardial infarct' gives a clear explanation to a fellow professional; to a patient, however, it is nonsense.

Jargon is not the same as gobbledegook, which is the use of long words and loose constructions which impress the writer but confuse the reader. Thus: *It has been observed that residents of domiciliary units constructed of a brittle and transparent nature are ill-advised to project into orbit small projectiles of geological origin* instead of *People in glass houses shouldn't throw stones.* As Brendan Hennessy writes: 'Gibberish or gobbledegook is likely to happen with professional people not used to writing for large audiences. They think the language of writing is altogether different from the language of speech; that, metaphorically, you dress in formal clothes to do it and choose a heavy pen'[3]. Phrases such as *Does this fit in with your perceptions?* and *Serious long-term medication is herewith predicated* are nothing more than a pompous and obscure way of saying *Do you agree?* and *You will have to take the pills for the rest of your life.* Yet such atrocities abound.

Scope of the book

The first surprise of the book may be that discussion of the use of language does not appear until Chapter 7. This is because the secret of successful writing hides below the water-line, at the preliminary stages of choosing the topic, the market, the research and the plan. Success depends on an even more basic question: should you be writing anyway? The next chapter, therefore, focuses on you as a writer. What do you expect to get from your labours? What can you offer, or – more important – not offer? How much time can you make available? Asking these questions and setting realistic goals from the answers is the surest way to long-term satisfaction.

These goals cannot be achieved in a vacuum, and Chapter 3 explains the world of publishing. If you want to become a good writer – which I define as someone whose words are regularly published with no substantial alteration – you must be able to answer three questions. What opportunities does the market offer? How does this market operate? And what is your place, as a writer, in it? Without this knowledge, any writing – however good the writer believes it to be – will remain undirected and unpublished.

After this brief foray into personality and product, the core of the book (Chapters 4-8) goes through the process of writing a feature article. These are articles of 600-2,000 words, which combine facts with comment. They are not scientific papers, nor are they news stories, which are shorter, factual items. I do not apologize for choosing this particular genre because many of the skills you will need for writing feature articles are essentially the same as you will need for other types of writing, and can be transferred easily. I have divided these skills into five main stages:

1) getting the brief,
2) collecting the material,
3) planning the article,
4) writing the article, and
5) doing the revision.

Some established writers may argue that their work goes straight into print, even though they do not follow these steps. That is not the point. I do not advocate 'writing by numbers', nor do I expect that those who ignore this process will be writing for the waste-paper basket. These stages are an attempt to bring order to a complex process, and to provide a framework which will ease nervous beginners into their first written article.

Once you have written your article, you must brace yourself for the next step, which is getting your article accepted. Editors are notoriously difficult people and the writer's path to publication is paved with cracked stones. Many of the problems stem from stereotyping: editors think that their contributors are arrogant and greedy while contributors think that their editors are greedy and arrogant. Chapter 9 proposes some solutions to this problematic relationship.

The final chapter will explain how you can develop your skills, get further training and, perhaps, turn to writing as a full-time career. The appendices list further reading, professional organizations, training opportunities, a code of ethics, a bluffer's guide to useful terms, and a selection of sub-editing marks.

Two basic principles

Two themes recur. The first, which has already surfaced, is that the actual writing, when empty coffee cups and angst pile up, is a relatively small part of the process. The real work, on which the success of an article depends, is done at a much earlier stage. Hence the importance of planning, of knowing what you are going to say, to whom and how. If you do this, you increase the chances of making your article work, and, incidentally, you will probably find that you have conquered writer's block, that demoralizing time when you spend long hours staring at a blank page or empty screen.

The second recurrent theme is that all successful writers share a particular attitude. Five elements are needed for successful communication to take place: a communicator (writer), a message (article), a receiver (reader), complete understanding by that receiver, and some kind of feedback (Figure 1.1). Most writing fails because it is written with the writer – and his or her superiors – in mind, or because the writer is over-concerned with the nuances of the message. Successful writers will view the transaction from the reader's point of view. This means putting your own needs out of your mind, and, if necessary, simplifying the message so that it can be understood. In other words, messages must be put across, not just put out, and the ultimate test is whether the reader understands. This point can never be too highly stressed.

Cynics will argue that the last thing we need is more writers in general and more medical writers in particular. We live in a world which is rapidly becoming immersed with bits of paper: the average professional will have dozens of pieces of paper landing on their desk each day. For doctors, with scores of unsolicited publications – not to mention instructions from authorities, learned articles from colleagues, letters to and from patients – clogging up their mailboxes, this must be much more.

Figure 1.1 Elements of communication

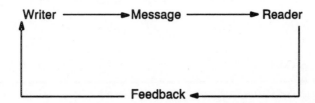

As we shall see in Chapter 3, the quantity of publications is generally beyond the individual's control. Yet the question of quality is not. A society that claims to be rational and democratic must support the free flow of ideas and information. The better these ideas and information, then the better our chances of moving forward, or at least not moving back. We will be presented with facts on which to base our opinions, and arguments that will stimulate our thoughts. At the same time we will be, in the broadest sense, entertained.

Doctors and other health workers have a duty to take part in this process. Their concern is with sickness and health, which is literally a matter of life and death to us all. They are one of the most highly trained groups of professionals, and have an education, outlook and experience that is extremely valuable. A world of ideas to which doctors did not contribute would be lopsided indeed.

Key points

1. This book assumes that writing skills can be taught. It will take the reader through five stages of writing a feature article: (a) setting the brief, (b) planning, (c) research, (d) writing and (e) revision.
2. Two themes will recur. (a) Writing is a small part of the process and planning is vital. (b) The ultimate test of good writing is that it is read and understood by the chosen audience.

2   Understanding the Writer

'*What you must on no account do is wait for inspiration*' – John Braine[4].

We all know someone who nearly wrote a novel. It would have been marvellous if they could only have found the time. Yet the only accomplishment that marks out a writer from the rest of the world is that the writer has made time. Whether the writings are published is beside the point.

Figure 2.1 Problems faced by writers

'I don't have enough time to write'	57%
'I wouldn't know how to start submitting an article'	50%
'I have so many ideas that I find it difficult to know which one to choose'	33%
'I have difficulty finding good ideas'	30%
'I find it difficult to stop researching'	30%
'My articles tend to be rejected'	20%
'I find I spend hours looking at a blank piece of paper'	17%
'My articles are too long'	17%
'I find writing easy'	17%
'Whenever I have written an article it has been changed considerably'	13%

(*Source: 30 doctors on one-day medical journalism courses*)

A questionnaire given to 30 doctors attending courses on medical journalism showed that more than half felt that their main problem was finding time (see Figure 2.1). Obviously this reflects the priorities they have chosen, but it is not the whole story. Any activity slips quickly down the list when you are not sure how to get started. This means that, if you are new to writing, you should not take yourself off to a darkened room 'to write'; you will end up with very little apart from balls of paper and depression. Instead, invest some time in asking yourself some basic questions. You will not need a desk to do this; scribbling on the back of an envelope in odd fragments of the day will do. Once you have answered these questions, you should be able to fit your new activity into your schedule.

Know what you want

Thousands of people write and thousands more try to do so. The rewards seem to be high. Admirers will cherish you for your wit and wisdom. Lucrative commissions will flow in and your bank manager will be amazed at the transformation of your finances. Your local paper will be full of photographs of your receiving prestigious awards for services to medical publishing, and conference organizers throughout the world, and particularly in the Caribbean, will send you first class return tickets for yourself and your partner. You might even make it onto *Question Time* or *Any Questions*.

Inevitably there is a down-side. Writing is in black and white. It will commit you, and those that you are writing about, to your statements in a way that speaking does not. Your opinions will often be seen to be critical, even if you didn't intend them to be, or, worse still, had taken great pains to disguise them. If you report the views of others, they will almost certainly accuse you of oversimplification. And, if you become a published author, others will feel uncomfortable because they did not do it first. The professional classes are not immune to jealousy.

It may not end in tears, but it could spoil a good meal. I remember one formal dinner at which the guest speaker, a distinguished medical writer, was 'buttonholed' by an eminent researcher, and publicly attacked for allegedly ruining the reputation of a colleague several years before. At least he was told of his offence, even though he couldn't remember it. Grievances tend to dwell in the minds of the aggrieved, and the medical establishment generally has far more subtle ways of dealing with 'offenders'. Because of this, one successful medical writer decided early in his career that he would not write for publication until he had become a consultant. The tone of his writing since has confirmed his sound judgement.

This does not mean that you should not write. But it does mean that, if you do, you should realize that you are putting your head above the trench, and will attract snipers. You should be aware of this risk, and decide in advance whether – or when – you wish to take it.

Motivation

One of the obvious rewards is the sheer pleasure of seeing your name in print. The power of this should not be under-estimated: I know of distinguished doctors who regularly cut out their articles and send them to their mothers. However, as argued above, high profiles have their dangers, and, if this is your only motive, I suggest that you consider some other competitive activity like hang-gliding or medical research, that will give you the fame you crave without the same danger to your career or personality.

Another reason for writing is to further your material interests, a motive to which, in post-Thatcherite Britain, we can readily admit. You may do this directly, by marketing articles which will earn vast sums of money, or indirectly, by using publication to bolster your reputation, career, practice or department. This is a straightforward reason, and success is easy to measure.

Professional people often say that they want to write because they have something to say. In itself this desire is harmless enough – the urge to influence others has as long a history as the urge to profit at their expense – and sublimating it into print is an innocuous way of meeting it. If you decide that this is your main motive for writing, you should ask three questions. What makes your opinions so special? What makes you think that others will be interested in them? And to what extent will you be willing to compromise in order to get them published and seen by others? The last question is particularly important: there is a huge gap between having something to say and being in a position to say it.

One of the pleasures of being a professional writer is that you are paid to find out things you would want to find out anyway. This should be coupled with a desire to tell others what you have found; this is the love of gossip in its more exalted sense of swapping information rather than assassinating personalities. Added pleasure may come from skilfully rocking boats without capsizing them, but be prepared for the shouts from passengers and crew.

Many writers say that they particularly enjoy the tussle between that blank piece of paper and themselves. Writing is an intensely personal activity, and one of the few areas in which people can exert full power over what they are doing (this power may rapidly evaporate once it reaches the editing stage, but that's for another chapter). One experienced doctor-writer summed it up when he told me that his main regret in his writing career had been that he had cashed his first cheque. He wished he had kept it framed, so that it could remind him forever of the intense satisfaction that publication had given him.

Some writers claim that they enjoy the process of writing, of sitting down and letting the words flow; others say that there is an inner demon which drives them to write. You can satisfy either need simply by sitting down and writing. There is nothing wrong with that, provided that you realize that your first priority is satisfying yourself rather than an audience, and that your chances of getting published rest on the unlikely event that the two coincide.

Motives are therefore important, because they will help shape the direction you choose. Anyone starting to write should understand their own; at worst this will avoid disappointment and, at best, will ensure a reasonable chance of becoming satisfied.

Skills

Do you enjoy meeting new people and listening to what they have to say, or would you prefer regaling them with your wit and wisdom? Such traits are as important as your motives, because they also suggest the direction you should take. The first category suggests reporting and interviewing; the second suggests opinion pieces or humour. They are both valid exercises, and each could lead to a successful writing career. The trick is to choose the one which suits you most.

As well as your skills, what specialist knowledge can you offer? You will be highly trained in medicine, but this merely puts you on a par with some 100,000 others. This doesn't mean that you should steer well clear of the subject, but that you should be careful about where you parade your expertise. A professor of gastroenterology with 40 years' experience might well be qualified to write in the journals as an expert on Crohn's disease, for instance, whereas a GP colleague of the same vintage may not. However, the GP would be qualified to write such an article in a local newspaper, and report on the views of experts for the specialist journals.

Dig a little deeper into your experience, perhaps by making a list of how you spend your time. Hobbies, such as stamp collecting or running up mountains, can be combined with your knowledge of medicine to capture a corner of the market. Don't write off the more mundane parts of your life, such as buying a flat overseas, dealing with officialdom, or struggling through rush-hour traffic. Good articles have been built from such unpromising subjects as using a dictating machine or filing a tax return. You are the undisputed expert in your own life, but be careful not to exceed your competence: there is a great difference between an article on how you fill in a tax return and one on the drawbacks of the current tax system. The first you are well-qualified to describe; the second you could write only with much research.

Logistics

Self-knowledge is not enough. You will also need the right equipment. This is not necessarily the most expensive (and I can write this from personal experience) but that with which you will be most comfortable. 'Don't chain yourself to a typewriter during the small hours if you would feel better writing in pencil before breakfast'[5].

You must have a place where you can write without interruptions, be it a spare bedroom, a shed in the garden, or even a seat on a train. Even in the train you will need a flat surface on which to write, and spread out your material. Don't stint on a seat: you will use it for long hours, and you will not want to risk back pain or, if you use a keyboard, repetitive strain injury.

You also need something to write with, which is not as banal a statement as it might seem. Some authors swear that a fountain pen gives them the only true rhythm for writing. The main disadvantage is that it usually requires the services of a typist to ensure that the final document has a fair chance of actually being read. More and more people use a word processor. These do make writing easier, though some writers have said that they have found that it panders to their innate verbosity. One dangerous innovation is the facility of moving text around after you have written something: this is no substitute for advance planning.

I have already mentioned the most important resource, which is time. Ask at an early stage how you can rearrange your priorities in order to leave some time for writing and all the other activities that go with it. You may find you can fit it into an odd hour, a lunchbreak perhaps, or a weekend. If you are coming up to retirement, you will be facing the prospects of large amounts of leisure: take the opportunity to fill them. Getting into a routine is far better than hoping to snatch the odd hour here and there. It is far more important to work regularly in short bursts than to rely on finding time when the muse strikes. That is one of the best ways of ensuring that the muse will keep well away.

Choose the market

The next chapter will look at the wide variety of publications, but it will help if you can narrow the field straight away. Where do you *not* want to be published? Some outlets you can dismiss at once: the tabloid press, for instance, will provide you with large audiences and large cheques, but at a price to your message and image that you may not wish to pay. Others may have a political stance with which you fiercely disagree, or deal with subject matter that you find boring.

At this stage your goal should be to have a general idea of the possible outlets for your work, and one or two definite publications that you can target. You will realize that there is an enormous amount of choice (see Figure 2.2), and the best advice is to concentrate on those publications which you read and enjoy. You will be familiar with them and will share their values. You will not find it hard to identify with their readers, because you are one.

Figure 2.2 Markets for medical writers

- **National press**: health pages, women's pages, other feature pages, Letters to the Editor, colour supplements, Doctor columns...
- **Local press**: Doctor columns...
- **Medical press**: opinion articles, clinical articles, reviews...
- **Scientific press**: papers, editorials, review articles, personal views...
- **Consumer magazines**: general articles on health, Doctor columns...
- **Specialist magazines**: articles on specialist subjects (e.g. health and computers)...
- **Newsletters**: general articles...

Set the goals

The final step is to start setting goals. These should be realistic. Rather than aim straight at the health page of a national newspaper why not start with a parish magazine? Instead of writing straight away, why not study a particular market, read a book on writing (finishing this one should count) or have published a Letter to the Editor. Goals should also be specific, with particular targets written down and kept wherever possible. You should set reasonable time limits, such as a year, and be progressive.

Put these goals on paper, and keep them (see Figure 2.3). Once you begin to meet them you will have made progress. What more could you ask?

Figure 2.3 Writer's checklist.

- Why do you want to write?
- What can you *not* offer?
- What *can* you offer?
- On which subjects do you wish to concentrate?
- For which audiences do you wish to write?
- Which publications will be most suitable?
- How much time do you want to spend on writing?
- What are your writing goals for the next 12 months?

Key points

1. Before starting, you should ask: (a) why you want to write, (b) what you can offer, and (c) what resources you need?
2. Use the answers to these questions to set yourself reasonable goals.

3   Understanding the Market

'Markets come before methods, and that is a message that beginners can be reluctant to learn', **Brendan Hennessy[6]**.

We are a nation of heavy readers. Each week, for instance, one man in 10 and one woman out of two reads a woman's magazine, according to the Periodical Publishers' Association[7]. The long-term trend is that this habit is increasing: the number of publications accepting advertisements went up from 3,800 in 1980 to nearly 6,700 in 1990. Some titles closed in the recession of 1991, but there is still more than one publication for every 10,000 men, women and children.

It's big business. The turnover from magazines in 1990 approached £2 billion, with £458 million spent on paper and printing, £281 million on staff, £74 million on postage, and £40 million on freelance contributions. This last figure, which would give 4,000 freelancers an annual income of £10,000 each, is good news because it shows how much the industry relies on outside contributors. Good editors will therefore seek them out, nurture and flatter them, and wherever possible poach them from their rivals. They will also be watching out for 'new' writers: that is, writers whose work they haven't seen before rather than those who have never been published.

To this extent, freelance contributors are in a seller's market, but they have to produce a satisfactory service. Writing talent is not enough. Editors, like doctors, have their own agendas, with such priorities as doing their job well (or at least not losing it), paying the mortgage and educating their children. They want contributors who will help them achieve these goals, and not start fruitless disputes over the exact placing of an apostrophe. In other words, they want professionals, not prima donnas.

You will almost certainly find this difficult to accept. Hours spent in a spare bedroom pouring out your love, time and intellect will make you form a close bond with what was just a blank piece of paper. But you must realize that your love child is about to be taken over. With luck, and some skill on your part, it is unlikely to be battered; but it will rarely stay exactly as you left it. What to you is part of your soul will become just one tiny component in this complex industry. If you are to become a professional writer, you must be prepared to accept the depressing fact that the importance of an article to *you* far outweighs its importance to anybody else.

Study the range

We use publications as we do our friends, coming back to them regularly for comfort and stimulation, and manipulating them in a way which serves our best interests. But, like any circle of friends, the range is limited. Go to any newspaper, or sift through any municipal rubbish dump, and you will see a vast range, from *Hair* and *Hello!* to *Catering Update*, from the comic *Viz* to *Puzzler* and the design engineering publication *Eureka*. As a writer, you must learn to see them as potential markets, not as litter.

But how can you make sense of them all? One way is to look at reference books such as *Willing's Press Guide*, the *Writers' and Artists' Yearbook* or *The Writer's Handbook*, (see Figure 3.1). But these tell only part of the story. To understand the market you need to know the five main ways in which publications differ: timing, format, distribution, ownership and readership. Each category holds important implications for the writer.

Figure 3.1 Entries from Willing's Press Guide, 1992

The Professional Nurse (1985), Ann Shuttleworth, Austen Cornish Publishers Ltd, Austen Cornish House, Walham Grove, London SW6 1QW *tel* 071-381 6301 *fax* 071-386 5482.
£22.50 p.a. M. Articles of interest to the professional nurse. *Length:* articles: 2500-3000 words; factsheets:1400 words; letters:250-500 words. *Payment:* by arrangement. *Illustrations:* line, colour, half-tone.

Pulse, Howard Griffiths, Morgan -Grampian (Professional Press) Ltd, Morgan-Grampian House, 30 Calderwood Street, Woolwich, London SE18 6QH *tel* 081-855 7777 *fax* 081-855 2406.
£72.00 p.a. W. Articles and photographs of direct interest to GPs. Purely clinical material can only be accepted from medically-qualified authors. *Length:* up to 750 words. *Payment:* £100 average. *Illustrations:* b&w, and colour photographs.

Quarterly Journal of Medicine (1907), *Publisher:* Oxford University Press, Pinkhill House, Southfield Road, Eynsham, Oxford OX8 1JJ; *Editorial:* Old White Hill, Tackley, Oxon.
£90.00 p.a. M. Devoted to the publication of original papers and critical reviews dealing with clinical medicine. *Payment:* none.

Timing

Publications have different rhythms, which are determined by how often they are published. Morning or evening newspapers deal with current events, though the immediacy of TV and radio means that they are moving towards more timeless analyses rather than 'hot news'. Weekly publications, such as local newspapers and professional magazines, still emphasize unfolding news events, but can do so because the stories they carry, or the 'angles' they put on them, are too localized to be published elsewhere.

Monthly publications are more leisurely. Their news sections usually contain the kind of news that can survive long lead-times between submission and publication. Shrewd editors of monthlies, and of publications which are even less frequent, will use their pages to make news rather than follow it. A dramatic example comes from the annual publication *Crockford's Clerical Dictionary* with its anonymous commentary on the state of the Church of England. In 1987 a highly critical preface caused a major storm, which culminated in the suicide of the supposed author and the axing of the anonymous preface.

Frequency of publication is important for the writer in three ways. First, as shown above, it will affect the type of subject you will choose. Second, it will affect your style of writing: generally the shorter the lead-time the tighter the copy. Third, it will affect the timing of your submission; a Christmas article, for instance, must be sent to a monthly while the summer flowers are still in bloom.

Distribution

The magazine industry distinguishes between consumer publications, which provide leisure-time information and entertainment, and business publications, which provide information on our working lives. Consumer publications are generally sold in shops and kiosks, unlike in the USA where most are sold by subscription and sent out by post. Their number in the UK has risen by about 40 per cent in the past 10 years, particularly in areas dealing with business and finance, country and regional matters, health and slimming, religion and politics – and angling. Figure 3.2 shows the most successful titles in terms of advertising revenue in 1989-90.

The business press (see Figure 3.2) has also grown, and particularly 'controlled circulation' publications or 'freebies', where the commercial advantage of a definable audience is judged to outweigh the benefits of having a cover price. These now have a combined annual circulation of more than 200 million readers. The specialist medical press is an

Figure 3.2 Top 12 titles by display revenue (1989-1990)

Consumer magazines:

Publication	Publisher	Feb 89-Jan 1990 (£m)
TV Times	IPC	46.5
Radio Times	BBC Magazines	38.2
Woman's Own	IPC	19.7
The Economist (UK)	The Economist	18.1
Country Life	IPC	17.1
Vogue	Conde Nast	15.5
Good Housekeeping	Nat. Magazine Co.	13.1
Woman	IPC	13.0
Cosmopolitan	Nat. Magazine Co.	12.9
Prima	Gruner and Jahr	9.7
Readers' Digest	RD Association	9.5
Ideal Home	IPC	9.5

(*Source: Media Register*)

Business magazines:

Publication (Paid or Controlled Circ.)	Publisher	Display revenue (£m)
Estates Gazette (P)	Estates Gazette (Reed)	10.1
PC User (CC)	EMAP Bus. Publishing	6.6
Pulse (CC)	Morgan-Grampian	6.2
Personal Computer World (P)	VNU Bus. Publicns.	5.6
General Practitioner (CC)	Haymarket	5.3
Estates Times (CC)	Morgan Grampian	5.0
Management Today (CC)	Haymarket	4.8
Farmers Weekly (P)	Reed Bus. Publishing	4.8
Computing (CC)	VNU Bus. Publicns.	4.8
Money Marketing (CC)	Centaur Communications	4.7
Doctor (CC)	Reed Bus. Publishing	4.6
Caterer and Hotel-keeper (P)	Reed Bus. Publishing	4.3

(*Source: Mediaweek / Media Monitoring Service*)

important part of this market, with an average turnover of about £50 million. Figure 3.3 shows that all but two of the top 10 highest spenders on display advertisements are pharmaceutical companies. Currently these concentrate on the GP market, which has a value about three times that for hospital doctors. Competition is particularly fierce, and actual readership is regularly monitored by surveys organized by Jicmars for GPs and Taylor Nelson for hospital doctors.

Figure 3.3 Top 10 business advertisers (1990)

Company	Category	Annual spend (£m)
Glaxo Laboratories	Medical	2.1
Allen and Hanburys	Medical	1.7
Pfizer	Medical	1.6
Merck Sharp and Dohme	Medical	1.2
Epson	Computing	1.1
Bayer UK	Medical	1.0
ICI Agrochemicals	Agriculture	1.0
Wellcome Foundation	Medical	1.0
Smith Kline and French	Medical	0.9
Janssen Pharmaceuticals	Medical	0.9

(*Source: Media Monitoring Service/ Media Week*)

The more successful a publication commercially, the greater the opportunities for freelance contributions. The thriving medical sector gives doctor-writers an obvious market. As Michael O'Donnell wryly remarks: 'One or two are first rate but the content of some reveal the strain their editors are under to find something to keep the advertisements apart.'[8]

Finances

Not all publications are run for profit. There is a whole range whose main aim is to communicate information, and are paid for by their sponsoring organizations. These newsletters have swept through the health services as fast as managers have discovered that their expensive computers can handle desk-top publishing.

They do provide a good market for writers, particularly those on the nursery slopes of the learning curve. In most cases they will pay little, but will provide good experience. In general, the more profitable the publication, the greater the fee. The mass-circulation magazines, including colour supplements, tend to pay several hundred pounds per 1,000 words, while controlled circulation publications will pay a little more than £100 per 1,000. There is another rule of thumb: the more prestigious the publication, the less it pays, on the grounds that writers should consider it a privilege to be published by them.

Ownership

A small number of companies or individuals own most of the major publications in this country. Research by the National Union of Journalists in 1988 showed how 10 companies controlled a wide variety of newspapers, magazines, book publishers, radio stations and television companies[9].

In reality, editors are no freer than the lunches they are said to enjoy. In a mercifully small number of cases, the proprietors take a close view of the contents. For instance, it is now widely discussed that the late Robert Maxwell often used the pages of the *Daily Mirror* to run flattering stories about himself. Generally, however, editors report to a publisher, whose main requirement from the editor is that they continue to attract readers without upsetting too many advertisers. Least fortunate are those who edit a publication controlled by a committee. This is not a good model, because committees multiply the need for ego-massage and tend to take the line of least resistance, ending up with the bland publishing the bland. This can lead to the *Pravda* effect, where a publication is so controlled that nobody believes anything it says.

You will soon learn how to define the political colours of a publication and how best to avoid the editor's pen. Often this can be done by careful rewording: *This is disgraceful*, can be softened through untraceable attributions, such as *Some critics say that this is disgraceful* or rhetorical questions like *Can this be right?*. Sometimes the conflict is best resolved by sending to another publication; one of the comforts of our system is that there is a huge range of publications, and, if you write well, you should be able to find a publisher somewhere.

Readership

All publications have a 'personality', which derives from each publication's readership and determines the type and style of articles. At one level this is easy to discover, and can be defined in stock sociological terms, such as gender, social class, geographical area, political slant, occupational group or spare-time interests. You will find some of these details by searching the handbooks, and by asking the advertising department to send its media pack which, for obvious reasons, will give an analysis of readers.

Yet this will not go far enough. It is said that *The Independent* appeals to literate independents, *The Times* to those who still believe in the concept of a top people's newspaper, *The Telegraph* to the commuting classes, and *The Guardian* to graduates in social sciences. The souls of those papers are relatively easy to discover, but, with medical papers, it gets harder. The difference between *Pulse* and *Nursing Times* is apparent, but what about *Pulse* and *Doctor*, or, harder still, *Pulse* and *General Practitioner*? How do you find out such subtleties?

The trick is to study each magazine carefully. What kind of articles does it carry? What kind of advertising? What are the interests revealed by the letters pages and other contributions from readers? What is the style of language: formal and a little pompous, or full of short sentences with short words? Is it written in a particular jargon, with a range of issues that constantly recur? Is there, perhaps, the slightest glimmer of a sense of humour?

Time spent in market analysis will not be wasted. The secret to successful freelancing is the same as that for producing a successful publication: finding a coherent audience and meeting its needs.

How publications work

Robert Day, Science Editor and Professor of English, tells the story of the pope who arrived in Heaven and complained when he discovered that a recently-arrived editor had much smarter accommodation. He was told that, while there were many popes in residence, this was the first time they had seen an editor[10]. Such abuse on an honourable profession is common. Frequent complaints include: 'Why have you cut my article in half?', 'How dare you desecrate my prose?' and (this usually said to a third party) 'That editor is so rude'. From the other side of the editorial desk, these complaints are seen differently: 'Why has he written 3,000 words when I asked for 800?', 'How can we use these incoherent ramblings?' and 'What makes him (rarely her, in my experience) always ring up on press day?'

Stereotyping abounds yet, as Arthur Plotnik comments in his useful little book on editing, 'editors need writers and even end up liking a few'[11]. The best way to end up being liked and published is to understand editors and the processes to which they are chained.

The role of the editor

Editors are responsible in law for all content, including advertisements, and therefore are the hub around which the great wheel turns, or grinds to a halt. On the one side they have to assuage the publisher, or members of the editorial committee; on the other loom the readers, whom they must amuse, titillate, inform and even offend, though not to the extent that they stop buying the publication. In between they have to massage a number of egos, which calls upon reserves of tact, charm and deviousness. They are directly responsible for the editorial staff, who form two main groups: those responsible for the intake of material, and those who have to turn this raw material into the finished product. Then there are those working for the same organization (or so the story goes) but not reporting to the editor, such as those responsible for advertisements, production and distribution (Figure 3.4).

Figure 3.4 The role of the editor

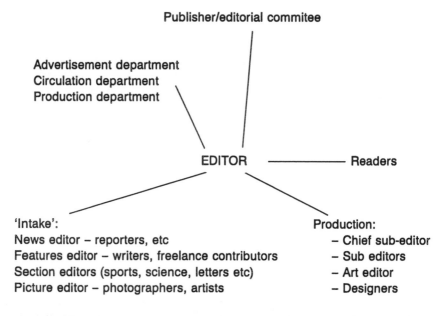

Successful editors must reconcile three different, and sometimes conflicting, aims. The first is to meet the financial targets, the second is to act within the political constraints, and the third is to attract as many readers as possible. Sometimes these come into conflict: editors of a house magazine, for instance, would attract many readers if they regularly reported the misdeeds of the executive committee; however, it is unlikely that they would stay in their post long enough to enjoy the plaudits. Alternatively, cutting back editorial expenditure by 50 per cent is likely to keep their management board extremely happy, though it is extremely unlikely that they will be able to keep their standards or readers, and in the long run the publication will fail, putting all out of work, bar the accountants.

Editors have a variety of powers, such as setting out the goals of the publication (unpopularly known as 'mission statements'), laying down policies on content and operation, holding regular debriefing meetings, hiring good staff, and raising standards through training. Perhaps the most important is their right to veto all articles and all page proofs. This gives them significant power over outside contributors: they can simply decline to have anything more to do with them.

The production cycle

Journalists, like doctors and other health professionals, try to do their job as best they can within budgets they always see as inadequate and facing a constant lack of time. But there is one important difference: time is not just short, it is punctuated with constant deadlines. If a publication is late, it loses revenue and readers. Deadlines are absolutes, and the need to meet them takes precedence over such luxuries as adding another fact or doing yet another check. And, as each deadline passes, another takes its place (Figure 3.5).

Figure 3.5 The editorial chain

PLANNING ⟶ COMMISSIONING ⟶ SUBMISSION OF MATERIAL ⟶

PROOF READING ⟵ SUB-EDITING ⟵ EDITORIAL APPROVAL ⟵

PAGE LAYOUT ⟶ PAGE PROOF APPROVAL

The cycle begins with the planning of each edition, when editors discover how much space is left for editorial use. Once the overall plan is agreed, the staff go to work to fulfil their allotted functions. The news editor assigns reporters according to a diary of coming events, while keeping some spare capacity for unexpected, or 'off-diary' stories. The features editor will choose from existing stock and commission some more. Others will select letters and write editorial comments. At the same time, the picture editor will make sure that there are appropriate illustrations.

As this material starts to come in, the editor, or a deputy, will decide if it can be used. Scientific publications have formalized this part of the process: original papers are sent to outside referees and finally selected or not at special meetings, sometimes called 'hanging committees'. Accepted material goes to the sub-editors, whose job is to ensure that it is accurate and well-written, legally safe and the right length. They also add the necessary embellishments, such as headlines and picture captions, to improve the chances of it being read.

The next part of the process takes many forms, thanks to the varying pace at which new technology is being introduced. The 'old' system of some 10 years ago called for manuscripts, or 'hard copy', to be sent to a typesetter, who produced a galley proof. Sub-editors would then design the page and send layout designs and corrected proofs to be turned into pages. The sub-editors would check the page proofs, trying to reduce extra charges by making textual corrections only when essential.

Desk-top publishing means that sub-editors can now do all these tasks themselves on their computer. They call up articles which have already been loaded into the computer by disk or through electronic means, such as modems. They edit this copy, and then design the page. This signals the end of many of the traditional printing crafts, though not everyone realizes that, while fewer printers are needed, more sub-editors are.

Approved pages are sent for processing, where they will be transformed into a photographic image, and the necessary illustrations and colour added. This will then be used to make the printing plate or plates (if in colour) from which the final image is made. Printing is an expensive business which ties up expensive plant for hours at a time. Each publication has its own time slot on the press, and, if it misses that slot, may find that it has to wait a considerable period of time before another can be found. This is another reason for keeping to deadlines.

The final stage consists of finishing the printed pages, by collating, cutting, binding and sorting them. The publication is ready to be distributed (see Figure 3.6). Meanwhile, back at the office, the editorial team are well into the next edition.

It is a long and complicated process, with many opportunities for error. Those involved in the process realize that they must concentrate on how many mistakes they spot rather than risk constant depression over the relatively few they miss. The mark of good editors is not that they make mistakes, because they will, but that they will make prompt and gracious amends once they have done so. Good contributors share this sense of proportion.

Figure 3.6 The publication process

ARTICLE, which is submitted to...

EDITOR'S OFFICE
which approves/rejects it and passes it to...

EDITORIAL / PRODUCTION DEPARTMENT
which corrects and amends it,
proofreads it,
oversees layout,
checks layout, and passes it to...

PROCESS DEPARTMENT
which turns it into photographic image,
adds colour and illustration,
and passes it to...

PRINTING HOUSE
which makes plates, which put the printed
image on the required number of copies,
and passes it to...

FINISHING DEPARTMENT
which trims, binds the copies
and distributes them.

Key points

1. The UK has a wide range of publications, which vary according to: (a) frequency, (b) distribution, (c) financing, (d) ownership and (e) readership. There are many opportunities for outside contributors, particularly in the specialist medical press.
2. To be a successful writer, you must understand the market. You must also see your role in context, as a relatively small part of a complex process.

4   Setting the Brief

'Don't start vast projects with half vast ideas', **Robert A Day**[12].

Life is full of potential articles. Patients come in with unusual conditions and interesting stories to tell. Governments and their representatives do silly things. New treatments conquer old diseases and new diseases spring up. There are riots, wars and famines, and amid it all we get collective hysteria over a group of musicians or a footballer. Meanwhile, real life goes on, with mortgages, examinations, bosses, employees, gardens, traffic jams, births, marriages and deaths.

We can all find topics which we, and other people, want to talk about, but turning them into articles is another matter. This explains the apparently contradictory results of the straw poll of doctors attending courses on medical journalism (see Figure 2.1, page 6) . One third said that they had so many ideas that they 'found it difficult to know which ones to choose' while another third said that they had 'difficulty finding good ideas.' Both are parts of the same problem.

The solution lies with a process which I call 'setting the brief', and which is the first of our five stages of writing a feature article. This chapter argues that you should be absolutely clear about your goals for each article before you start. As your reputation grows, editors will often define this goal for you, though, bearing in mind the dictum that 'an editor is someone who knows exactly what he wants but isn't quite sure', you will almost certainly have to do some refining. Until you reach this stage, you will have to set the brief yourself.

From subject to idea

Your aim is to produce an idea for an article that readers – and editors – will find interesting: 'Write about what other people want to know rather than about what you happen to know,' advocates Brendan Hennessy[13]. This begs the question: what do people want to know?

Health is a popular subject, according to a survey published in *Nature* which asked 2,009 British adults their opinions on six subject areas. The most popular was new medical discoveries (with 49 per cent 'very interested'), followed by new inventions and technologies (39 per cent), new scientific discoveries (38 per cent), sport (28 per cent) new films (17 per cent) and politics (16 per cent). Out of 13 sample headlines, the most popular was *Heart disease our own fault, claim experts*[14].

This sheds light on the broad subjects of interest, but it does not explain why some items in each subject area are apparently more interesting than others. A former colleague used to claim that there were only four health stories: first, patients will suffer unless doctors get more (or, in the current version, administrators get less); second, new treatment gives hope; third, old treatment causes cancer; fourth, jogger's nipple – the novelty story. To this I would now add one more: fifth, TV star fights fatal disease. Cynical perhaps, but like all good cynicism there is an element of truth.

A more serious analysis would include the following elements. An interesting story will be timely: relevant to *now*, and preferably *new*. It will also be close to the reader, which explains why five deaths on the M1 will get more space in a newspaper than 50 drownings in a ferry accident in Latin America. It will deal with significant amounts: a £1 saving is not a talking point, but £1m would be. It will affect people, preferably those with whom the reader can identify or a 'household name'. Finally, it may have an element of surprise and conflict: the fact that a Tory MP goes into a private hospital will not detain a reader long, but, if a Labour spokesman on health is discovered having done so, that becomes a talking point.

Of course, this does not help you find those stories in the first place. If you don't have any ideas, and the chances are you won't, then you will have to find them, which is easier than it sounds. Take a broad subject and brainstorm. More prosaically, write down the subject in the middle of a piece of paper, and then write down the thoughts that occur to you.

Take, for instance, sabbaticals. It's a rather dry subject, as it stands – but can be developed in many directions (see Figure 4.1). We can soon find several interesting questions, which meet many of the criteria mentioned above. Are sabbaticals a waste of time? Should the NHS introduce them?

Would they help doctors avoid 'burn-out' and therefore produce a better service? If they are introduced, how should people use the time – by reducing their golf handicap, by going to the Third World or by following an Open University course in business management? Are there any psychological or medical implications? Is the whole idea too expensive?

Figure 4.1 Brainstorming

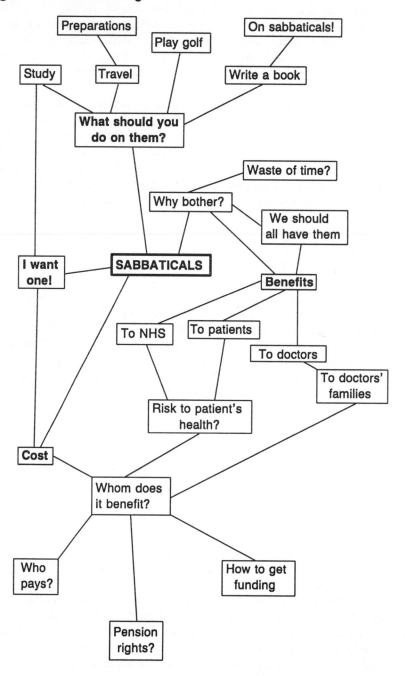

What started as a single broad subject has now spawned a number of ideas, and it is easy to choose other themes and develop them in this way. Look out for subjects that arouse interest. Note them down: there is one thing worse than not having ideas – and that is having good ideas and forgetting them. As you become more accomplished, they will start to appear, but not always when you expect them. Many established writers carry a notebook, so that they can preserve their good ideas long enough to start working on the next stage, which is refining them into a definite proposal.

Working on the idea

This is the time to meet the 'honest serving men' attributed to Rudyard Kipling. These are the simple but effective questions: Who? Where? What? When? Why? and How? Others have since added two more: Why me and So what? These ideas, inflated by jargon, seem to form the basis of much modern management theory, but the Victorian simplicity of Kipling's version makes a useful litany. They are questions that can be usefully asked at most stages of writing and submitting an article.

Where?

Once you have a possible idea, try to match it to a market. Here again a brief brainstorm should produce an adequate list. To develop the idea of sabbaticals, the argument that all doctors should have them every five years could suit one of the medical newspapers. The medical editors of the *Independent* or *Guardian* might well buy an angry article on how 'burnt-out' doctors should have three months off every five years for the sake of their patients. Twist it around slightly for the *Health Service Journal*: sabbaticals would save money for the NHS because they would reduce the number of 'burnt-out' doctors. A business magazine might be interested in what health precautions should be taken before going on a sabbatical, or *Punch* might take a whimsical piece on how patients should club together and send their GP to foreign parts – or why GPs should club together to send some of their patients even further away. The possibilities, if not endless, are plenty.

Why?

Now that you have linked your idea with a possible market, see if you can destroy it. Will you be saying anything interesting? You may think so, but will others agree? Will you be saying anything new, or is it just an old treatment of an old idea? Is the idea based on a false premise? Can you actually prove it? Does it meet any of the elements of a 'good story' mentioned above?

Don't necessarily reject the idea if the answer is no to any of these. Try altering it slightly to take account of your objection, or match it to a different market. For instance, readers of *Doctor* are unlikely to be interested in the fact that medical academics are coming back from their sabbaticals with all kinds of revolutionary ideas; readers of the *Times Higher Education Supplement* might.

How?

If the idea has passed the 'Why' test, ask which broad approach you will take to gather the necessary material. There are many different ways of writing articles: factual or opinionated, serious or funny, informative or provocative (see Figure 4.2). Choose in advance which style will be best for your subject, your market and your abilities. In this way you can adopt the right style from the start.

Figure 4.2 Types of articles

News	There has been a new development concerning sabbaticals.
Backgrounder	This is how the new development came about.
Situationer	All you need to know about sabbaticals.
Interview	All the greatest living expert knows about sabbaticals.
Profile	All you need to know about the greatest living expert on sabbaticals.
Service	How to organize a sabbatical.
Personal	This happened to me on my sabbatical.
Humour	This funny thing happened to me on my sabbatical.
Think-piece	What I think of sabbaticals.
Commentary	What other people think about sabbaticals.
Polemic	I am going to provoke you into thinking about sabbaticals.
Leader/edit- orial	What my editor thinks about sabbaticals.

Some practical problems could appear. It is no use, for instance, proposing an interview with the world's greatest living expert on the medical implications of sabbaticals if he lives in California (as indeed he will) and you cannot afford the fare, or the telephone call. Again, if there is a problem, try approaching the article another way. Perhaps the second greatest living expert lives in Swindon.

When?

Consider also when the article is likely to be published? Will it be timely? There is no point writing an article on Christmas for the summer, and every point in writing one on summer holidays to appear just after Christmas when the brochures appear. Is someone else likely to write it, in which case can you get yours in first? If not, don't bother. Has it got a topical angle, or is it likely to end up as a 'yo-yo' article, going into the schedule at the beginning of each production cycle, and coming out shortly afterwards when a more urgent story appears? If this looks likely, put in a topical 'peg', like an anniversary or a conference, which will give it a definite shelf-life.

Whatever the urgency of the article, you should give yourself a deadline. If you don't, you may find it hard to finish.

Why me?

Are you the right person to write the piece? Don't be put off if you are not an expert: they are often the worst people to explain complex ideas to those who have not studied at their feet. The fact that you can understand and interpret is ample qualification. On the other hand, if you are not an expert do not write as if you are. As advocated in Chapter 2, stick to your areas of competence.

So what?

Do you still want to proceed, or have you been tempted down a path of unutterable trivia? If so, now is the time to cut your losses and think up another idea.

Set the brief

You should now be ready to define your brief formally. For example: *A 900 word article by next Friday for* Medeconomics *on how to finance sabbaticals*. Or: *A 900 word article before the end of the month for* Punch *on how patients should finance sabbaticals*. The more specific the better. Note how two changes (*Medeconomics* to *Punch* and the insertion of *patients*) alter the article considerably. Such changes can be subtler still: instead of *finance sabbaticals* put *finance my sabbatical*. These are two separate articles and would need two different approaches.

Make sure you limit it to one idea. An article on *...how to finance* *sabbaticals and whether GPs should have them tax deductible and hospital doctors should be able to apply for special grants...* is going to give you problems from the start. It may well be too broad for the space available. More important, you will find it impossible to construct a coherent argument. Either reduce your ideas to one, which will force you to decide which is the most important, or split them up into several different articles.

Being able to summarize in one sentence the theme of your article will pay many dividends when you come to the next four stages. You may have to amend your brief in the course of your research, but having it clearly fixed in your mind at this stage will help you to focus on gathering the material you now need to turn 35 words into 1,000.

Key points

1. The first stage in writing an article is to have a clear and simple view of the kind of article you intend to write. This stage is called 'setting the brief'.
2. A good brief consists of: (a) market, (b) length, (c) deadline, and (d) a single clear idea.
3. The idea should be tested with the following questions: Where? Why? How? When? Why me? and So what?

5   Doing the Research

'*Spell a man's name incorrectly and he will be deeply hurt, because it's all his own, and he will spread the news around*', **Leslie Sellers**[15].

As a doctor you should have no fears about research. You will have endured at least seven years of scientific training, and could be forgiven for feeling that, in this chapter at least, you are on safe and familiar ground. Be careful. This assumption could be dangerous, tempting you down pleasant but barren by-ways, wasting time and energy, and ending with a muddled and rejected article – or no article at all.

There is a world of difference between the research needed for a piece of writing and the research needed for a piece of science. Science, and its 'kissing cousin' diagnosis, assumes that it is edging towards The Truth; scientific papers reflect this attitude and are chosen to be right rather than to be read. Other types of writing, however, set their sights rather lower.

Their goal is to inform, stimulate and entertain, not necessarily in that order. They do this by reporting facts or opinions, or by making original, preferably controversial, observations. They realize that their words will be worthless unless they are read and understood. Quite sensibly, these writers avoid seeking The Truth in 1,000 words, but they do try to ensure that they are *not wrong*. The difference between 'describing The Truth' and trying to be 'not wrong' may be a fine distinction, but it has important implications: it means that those who are used to writing science must accept the limitations of their new activity. This does not mean lower standards, but it does mean different standards. Experienced scientists should resist the temptation to set about researching an article in the same way as they would research a learned paper. It would be a waste of time, and would produce an over-complicated and unreadable article.

The trick is to research the brief, not the subject. If it has been clearly stated, a number of questions will arise. For instance, a feature writer researching an article arguing that *a limited drug list is a waste of time* would not start by looking up all the references on the subject, but would list the questions he or she would need to make this point. These could include: (1) what is the present situation?, (2) what is wrong with it?, and (3) what needs to be done to make it better? A slightly different brief would inspire a different set of questions: if the brief were for an article arguing that *a limited list does not save money*, the obvious questions would be: (1) how much does it cost? (2) how much does it save?, and (3) is a limited list worth it?

This saves time and produces a more readable article without necessarily losing important facts. What you now need to do is decide how you will gather the information.

Sources

Any theme can be tackled in a number of ways. Take, for instance, an article on cervical smears. It could be a report of a new study. It could be a review of the literature (though, even such 'trips round the block' should come up with some original angle, either of interpretation or analysis). It could set out a personal view, report a conference, interview a patient (perhaps someone who has waited for months to receive her results) or be a first-person account by, say, a doctor who has been through the process and wishes to argue that it is excellent, or dehumanizing.

The brief and the chosen method of research are closely intertwined. In some cases, the brief may even state what research will be used (for instance, *an interview with...*). Once you have a broad idea of how you will gather your material, ask some more questions. What is the minimum information you need to sustain your argument, prove your point or describe a situation? Where can you find this information? What is the most efficient way of getting it? And will the resulting article be accurate and balanced?

Scientific studies

Hectares of good trees have been devoted to the proper way of carrying out scientific studies. Fortunately for the trees that remain, this is beyond the scope of this book. Suffice it to say that the proper place for a scientific study is a journal (see Chapter 10 for some brief comments on the subject). However, sometimes a quick survey will add considerably to a non-scientific article. There is nothing wrong with that, provided that the methods are clearly stated, so that readers can interpret the results accordingly.

Personal experience

Many articles are constructed on the strength of personal experience, or what is called 'off the top of one's head'. These could include a specific anecdote ending with a general message, or a succession of opinions. If you choose to write in this way, take special care that you only write about what you know and check any facts you use, however sure you are that you have remembered them correctly. If you are writing about patients, remember confidentiality and ensure that they are not recognized. In some cases you may have to change some details, such as age, gender or occupation.

Written material

Written sources must be approached with care. First, mastering all the relevant literature can take up huge amounts of time. Second, the writing style will rarely translate into pithy quotations. Third, they may be wrong. I worked for one magazine which printed in good faith a figure purporting to be the number of teenage drug addicts in London. It was quickly pointed out to us that this figure was greater than the number of teenagers in the capital and we ran a correction in the next issue. Nevertheless the 'fact' acquired a momentum of its own, and for months we received cuttings from publications all over the world which perpetuated this false figure. However quick the correction, it is rarely fast enough to head off these epidemics of misinformation.

However, written sources are suitable for background reading, but for most newspaper and magazine articles, the best source of information is the interview.

Interviews

Interviews will give you up-to-date information and alert you to errors in written sources. If you choose with care, you will gain access to an expert who will have done most of the leg-work for you. He or she will provide you with lively quotes, because people speak less pompously and more vividly than when they write. You will also have the chance to ask further questions, which will be specific to your brief.

Make sure that your sources are qualified to talk about the subject, and that you balance their views with opposing views. You can find out who is likely to give an opposite opinion by looking at the literature, by asking people in the know, by going to reputable third parties such as professional organizations, or even by asking the interviewee. You will not need much information to flesh out your brief, so it is the quality, not the quantity, of interviews that is important.

Before each interview try to find out about the subject; that should avoid starting off from a position of embarrassment. (I once heard of a cameraman who was trying to relax his subject. 'What do you do?' he asked. 'Minister of Health' came the reply.) Structure the interview, not by working through a long list of questions, but by working out three or four main areas you wish to explore. By all means write down a number of questions, but use it as a checklist at the end of the interview rather than as a prompt sheet throughout.

Establish the ground rules at the start. Tell the interviewee what the story is about – sometimes you may find it tactful to be vague – and for which publication you are writing. Assume that the subject realizes that he or she will be quoted. If they are clearly unhappy about that, negotiate. You may agree that the interview is non-attributable, in which case you can use the information but not the source. (Thus: *informed sources say...* or *experienced researchers argue...*) Never agree that the whole interview should be off-the-record: this would be a waste of time because you will not be able to use the information; as a last resort agree that certain parts will be off-the-record, provided that the interviewee makes this clear before saying them.

Interviews do go wrong, with the subject refusing to answer carefully-prepared questions or, more usually, telling you what you do not need to know. Control the interview, keeping to the issues you have picked out in advance. This may require drastic measures, like staring into space or picking your nose, but generally good questioning will suffice. Beware asides, even if they do sound interesting.

Finally, at the end of each interview, use your checklist. You should then ask three vital questions: (1) 'Do you have anything further to add?', (2) 'Should I talk to anyone else?' and (3) 'How can I contact you again?'. The first can yield unexpected delights ('Well, it so happens that I have the Victoria Cross and was the first man with one leg to swim the channel'); the second can unearth promising sources; and the third can be invaluable in checking facts or finding out further information. Most interviewees will not see these questions as a mark of failure, but will be impressed by your thoroughness.

Other senses

These are much neglected. Good articles are made up not only of the words that people speak, but also of what they did, what they looked like, and how they reacted. Vividness comes from using details gleaned from using senses other than hearing: touch (did the interviewee keep stroking his ear or your leg, for instance?), or smell (was there a smell of tobacco in the health fanatic's room?), or even taste (did his comments match the acidity of the raspberries you were eating at the time?). Such details, used skilfully, lift an article out of the ordinary. But beware jumping to conclusions: an amber liquid in a whisky glass may be ginger ale not Black Label, and the drinker may be offended if you get it wrong, particularly if the interview has taken place over breakfast.

Conferences

Conferences can be a useful and rapid way of gathering information. If the organizers know what they are doing, they will have done much of your work for you by gathering together several experts on a particular subject.

Again, make your intentions clear. If you are planning to report what is said, you should make this clear to the organizers, particularly if you have registered in the normal way. Make sure that the facts you report are correct: seeing a stack of figures flashed on a screen in a darkened room is one of the worst ways of getting information. Don't be afraid to buttonhole the speaker afterwards, though you might have to make clear that he or she was speaking after the conference.

Conferences can be reported in a number of ways. The most commonly seen in the paramedical press is the news report, in which one aspect of a long speech is picked out and developed, often outside the conference. A second way, common among inexperienced writers, is the conference report which is structured along the lines of the conference itself: *After an excellent lunch of chicken wings and salad, Professor Calabrese spoke of the effects of... .* This approach may satisfy the speakers' desires to see their name in print, but will rarely make a serious point; like all shopping lists, it will appeal only to the serious shoppers. My preferred solution is to use the conference as a resource, not a timetable. Listen carefully and then come up with one theme for the article; use information and quotations from the various speakers to support *your* argument. This is selective, but stimulating. It is not always appropriate; if in doubt ask your commissioning editor – *before* the conference.

Press conferences

These are events organized by those who want to make the news, in which they generally make a statement to invited journalists and then invite questions. At the same time they will issue a press release, intended to steer journalists towards the story that they wish to put out. This doesn't always work: if a better story comes along, don't hesitate to risk the wrath of the PR organizers and use it. It has been said in public.

Unfortunately, some people cannot resist the temptation to use press conferences as a platform for themselves, making long statements rather than asking brief questions. If this happens, use the 'dead time' to work out your story, and confine your questions to what you need to write it. Be aware that asking questions will show your hand: if you think you may have an exclusive angle then try to stand it up afterwards, in private.

Organizing material

Recording

The rise of the Japanese tape recorder now means that everyone has a simple way of ensuring an accurate record of proceedings. But this is not a perfect solution. In conferences, it may not be possible to get close enough for good sound. In interviews, the sight of a running tape may frighten the subject into platitudes. Also, mechanical objects have mechanical breakdowns, and nothing can be worse than coming away from a good interview to discover that the tape hasn't been running. One colleague once discovered that the whole of his exclusive interview with the Secretary of Health had been lost. Fortunately he managed to get another interview, which gave him much better information. Such second bites are rare.

Tape recorders can also be extremely time-consuming. Few can resist the temptation to let them do all the work, which means that they then have to listen to everything again. At best this doubles the research time. Look upon the tape recorder as a back-up. Take notes. Make some kind of mark in the margin when someone makes a statement that you think you can use.

Shorthand does help, but most interviewers can quickly develop their own type of speedwriting. Make sure you label clearly where each piece of information comes from; with interviews this can develop into a useful habit; checking with each subject the proper spelling of their name and title is a non-threatening start to an interview, and sends the message that you care about getting facts right.

Retrieval

Some people are not satisfied unless they can go back after an interview and type up their notes; this is a waste of time. It is better to go through your notes underlining the bits you expect to use or jotting them down on another piece of paper. Read your notes as soon as you can because this will help you interpret them correctly. Don't tear them up as soon as you have written the article: you may need them for a rewrite, but, more important, you will certainly need them if those you interview question your version of events. In such cases, keep calm; if you have a good note you can often prove that you are right, and that their memory is faulty. Even after the article has been published, it is good practice to store away all source material, carefully labelled.

But this is moving ahead. At the moment you will have many thousands of words in your notebook which you now have to boil down to about 1,000. How do you go about this painful process?

Key points

1. The aim of the 'research stage' is not to find out all there is to know about a subject, but to provide enough information to fill out your brief. Try to be 'not wrong', rather than to discover 'The Truth'.
2. There are many ways of gathering this information, such as interviews, observations, conferences and press conferences. Which one you choose will depend on the brief you set yourself.
3. All information should be clearly recorded and subsequently stored.

---

6   Planning

'There is no substitute for a detailed plan', **John Whale**[16].

I once heard the American author Arthur Hailey (*Hotel, Airport* etc) explain the technique that netted him enough to live in some style in the Bahamas. Each book took him three years. The first he spent immersing himself in the subject and the third in actual writing. For the whole of the second year he planned the book's structure.

Surprising perhaps, but when writing fails it is usually because of its structure, not its style. Readers are only too happy for an excuse to stop reading one document and get on to one of the many others queueing up for their attention. The quickest way to lose that interest is to make the writing difficult to follow, by lurching off into unannounced byways, by presenting an indigestible feast of information, or by having a plan so sophisticated that only you can understand it.

The solution is simple: (1) work out a plan, and (2) stick to it. The first takes time, and a little deferred pleasure as you resist the temptation to start writing. It can be worked out on any piece of paper, from a snow-white sheet of foolscap to a wine-stained napkin. Writing the brief at the top of the page will focus your mind on your brief. If you decide, even at this stage, that you must alter it, do so, but make sure that it still consists of one idea; don't just tack on new ones.

Sticking to the plan is harder. It is as inevitable as a broken-down photocopier before a meeting that you will have far more information than you need. A one-hour interview will probably yield about 5,000 words. Therefore a 1,000 word feature based on three interviews will force you to discard 14 words out of 15. Some of these words will be good ones, containing provocative ideas, significant new information, or nuances that an expert would appreciate. However, squeezing them in is the quickest way to destroy the clarity of your brief. Your priority must be structure, not content.

The opening

Many articles stand little chance of being read because their first few paragraphs are dull. Sometimes writers will give a summary of what they are about to say. Sometimes they will start with a trail of boring words, as in: *The ways and means sub-committee of the general purposes committee decided at their meeting last week...* . Sometimes they will recite a series of platitudes; this is throat-clearing, which allows experienced sub-editors to carry out apparent miracles by lopping off the first paragraph.

Sally Adams, writing in a handbook for magazine journalists, lists five different ways of starting a feature article: (1) telling a story, (2) describing a scene, (3) using a quotation, (4) stating facts, and (5) giving an opinionated pronouncement[17]. We should take it one stage further: a story should be interesting, a description should be vivid, a quotation should be strong, facts should be intriguing and an opinion controversial. An article which starts: *Mr Justice Brown fined an Ealing man £500 in the High Court yesterday after pleading guilty to a charge of grievous bodily harm...* is unlikely to detain us long. However, this story would: *A police inspector who used a carrot to hit a Roman Catholic priest over the head was fined £500 in the High Court yesterday*. Same story; higher readership.

The important thing is to remember the purpose of the first few paragraphs. Do not be misled by the genteel implications of the term 'introduction', which calls up an image of someone making polite preliminary remarks to an attentive listener. This is not the function of the opening. Despite what you may have been taught at school, it is not a summary either; your readers, unlike your teachers, are not being paid for reading your prose. Its purpose is brutal: to attract the reader's interest so that he or she will want to start – and finish – the piece of writing. It is where your victim will be hooked, or left to swim out of range.

Consider these three introductory paragraphs from one edition of *The Independent's* Health Page (January 29, 1991):

'In many respects it is easier and less uncomfortable to have leukaemia than eczema...' (Mark Handscomb).

'Jill is physically disabled and unable to walk more than a few steps at a time. She has recently developed a heart condition, which makes it almost impossible for her to visit her doctor's surgery. Every time she needs treatment, he has to visit her at home. He does not have the resources to provide this service, however, and, as his legal right, has struck her off his list of patients.

'Jill telephoned her local Community Health Council for help. 'We're trying to find another doctor who will take Jill on,' said Josephine Barry-Hicks, Ealing's CHC secretary for the past 12 years. 'But if we can't, she'll be allocated to different GPs for three to six months each. The Family Health Services Authority has the power to insist a doctor takes on a patient for part of the year. We've got several cases like this...' (Anne Wiltsher).

'This is a story of sex, fear and money. It is about a new treatment for an embarrassing problem which could prove a money spinner in the new commercial National Health Service...'(Jeremy Laurance).

They all have one thing in common: they grab the reader's attention and set up a dynamic that will only be satisfactorily answered at the end of the article. Mark Handscomb starts with an outrageous idea: how can a dermatological complaint possibly be as bad as leukaemia? Anne Wiltsher tells a personal story, going from a particular incident to her general subject (Community Health Councils). Jeremy Laurance achieves the remarkable feat of using three of the most emotive words in the English language in the first sentence. He then sinks the hook deeper still by posing an intriguing paradox: a chance to make money for the NHS. We want to know his conclusion.

Conclusion

Getting out of an article should be easier than getting into it. We no longer have to keep readers interested; they are already there. All we have to do is leave them with our intended message. This is where our brief should come into its own: if it is a good one, all we have to do is answer the question it poses. This can be done by making our own judgment; by quoting somebody else's (this has the advantage of allowing you to be provocative without committing yourself); by referring back to a point made in the opening, and elaborating on it; or by giving one final provocative twist. You should not regurgitate what you have already said, or simply put down your pen. The final paragraph is not an ending or a summary, but a conclusion.

In the articles mentioned above, Mark Handscomb was writing about a Chinese woman doctor's cure for eczema. He concludes by quoting the opinion of a consultant dermatologist who refers patients to her:

> ' "This is the most promising treatment for eczema since the advent of corticosteroids 40 years ago. What is surprising is that we were so unaware of the benefits that this kind of treatment can achieve" '

Ann Wiltsher's article examines the changes that could restrict the useful work of the Community Health Councils. She also concludes with a quote, but has a pleasant symmetry by quoting Mrs Barry-Hicks, whom she quoted in the opening. She also has a deft twist, by pointing out that Community Health Councils are not themselves above blame:

> 'Nobody at my regional health authority really knows what I'm doing. I can do what I like as long as I don't bop the clients or put my fingers in the till or behave in a bizarre way that gets into the newspapers. I'm not saying that there should be a rigid bureaucracy, but there should be minimum standards that should be checked and enforced.'

The theme of Jeremy Laurance's article is how the new technique of heat-shrinking prostates could be a money spinner for the NHS, because the procedure will probably need repeating every few years. He concludes with a provocative question:

> 'In the NHS of the nineties, fashions will change as rapidly in Britain's hospitals as on the Paris catwalks. It will mean more choice for family doctors and patients. But will it mean better value?'

Readers now have enough information to make up their own minds.

Development

Having decided on the beginning and the end, the next problem is working out how to get from one to the other. As in the research stage, focus on the brief, not the subject. Temptations will appear: fantastic beasts will rear up out of the undergrowth and juicy red herrings swim constantly into view. Again, concentrate on the purpose of your expedition, not the subject or, indeed, individual objects.

More specifically, keep it simple, keep it balanced and keep it logical. As a general guide, allow no more than one major point every 300 words. Do not expand any single point to the detriment of others. And make sure that they flow on easily from one to the other. Don't be afraid to use link words, such as *However, The next point, At the same time* and, as in this paragraph, *More specifically.* You may find it tedious to rake these out of your repertoire, but they will provide the reader with a smooth passage.

Let us now return to the suggested article on how making patients wait for their consultations can rebound on doctors. A possible structure could be as follows:

BRIEF: *An article for* BMA News Review *showing how making patients wait for their consultations can rebound on doctors.*

INTRODUCTION: Personal account of waiting around in a clinic which started one and a half hours late.

DEVELOPMENT:
(1) As a psychiatrist, time is a major issue;
(2) It is 'not on' for me to be late:
    (a) punctuality builds up a relationship of trust,
    (b) being on time shows that I care;
(3) Is being a psychiatrist different from being a physician or a surgeon?
(4) There is no real difference:
    (a) doctors seeing private patients can do it,
    (b) the relationship is just as important as in psychiatry;
(5) So why does it happen?
    (a) doctors see patients as inferior,
    (b) doctors treat patients as objects (more likely explanation)

CONCLUSION: There is no excuse for keeping patients waiting: good organization and politeness cost nothing.

The structure is clear and easy-to-follow. Each part can now be 'fleshed out' with supporting evidence. Each transition can be linked, with phrases such as *First..., Second..., One explanation put forward...,* and *It is more likely, however....* . The article seems publishable, which in fact it was (Figure 6.1).

Figure 6.1 The waiting game

Sarah Newth (in *BMA News Review*) takes a close look at how making patients wait for their consultations can rebound on doctors.

Recently I had an appointment at an out-patients which was reminiscent of an old practical joke – the one where the newest apprentice is sent to the stores for the long stand. I had to wait a couple of hours. At least I had a chair so that I could sit and think about writing an article about waiting – but that did not make it any funnier.

I suppose I was lucky. My 9 o'clock appointment was my own, not one of those in which everyone is told to come at the same time. So when the clinic eventually started, one and a half hours late, I was seen quickly.

I am a psychiatrist who works with children and families so, for me, being on time is a big issue. Patients are often late and this may be for a variety of reasons: they may not really want to come; they may be angry with me but unable to put it into words; or they may simply be disorganized, which could be why they are seeing me in the first place. These reasons are important and need to be addressed as part of therapy.

For me to be late seeing them is decidedly not on. If I say 10 o'clock, then I have to see them at 10 o'clock. If I say that we finish at 10.30, then that is when we finish. *It is part of the structure you have to set up,* within which a relationship of trust can be built. If I don't do as I say, how can I be trusted to listen?

Being on time shows that I care. People have to make arrangements to visit a doctor. They have to take time off work, arrange babysitting and catch buses. Sometimes, they lose money if they miss work, or even their jobs. Keeping them waiting and making them late implies that I am not bothered about that part of their lives. It also implies that I do not respect them, that their time is less important than mine.

Perhaps being a psychiatrist is different to being a physician or surgeon. Giving people time is as much a tool of my trade as a scalpel is to a surgeon. When I sat in out-patients waiting, I felt angry and frustrated. I also found myself making excuses for the doctor I was waiting for: maybe he or she was busy, held up in theatre, seeing an emergency. By the time the clinic started, I was almost apologizing for being there.

Thinking about it now, *there is really no difference between other doctors and me.* Doctors seeing private patients can suddenly become organized enough to see them on time, because they pay for it. They are also given individual appointments, not group ones.

Second, the relationship between patient and doctors is just as important in a medical consultation as a psychiatric one. A patient who sits in out-patients for hours becomes more and more anxious. He is rightly going to feel that he is getting second best and will be suspicious of his treatment as a result.

Trust and respect, which are so important in my work, are basic human values which form the foundation of any relationship. Why should the doctor-patient relationship be treated any differently?

One explanation put forward is that *some doctors actually see patients as inferior beings* whose lives matter less than theirs. Perhaps they see patients' illness as a sign of weakness or as their fault? Putting them to a certain amount of inconvenience could be their way of showing disapproval.

It is more likely, however, that the way we are educated to regard patients as cases means that we don't even think about it at all. We are brought up thinking that it is a bad thing to become emotionally involved with patients, so we treat them as objects.

Whatever the reason, doctor-knocking is a fashionable occupation. Litigation is increasing and costing your profession a lot of money. *Good organization and politeness cost nothing.* In fact, it could even make patients feel so much better that they no longer wish to sue. It gives a new meaning to the saying 'time means money'.

BMA News Review (February 1988).

Key points

1. Make a plan and stick to it. Writing is about taking decisions, and some of the hardest concern what to leave out.
2. An article has three elements:(a) the introduction or opening, (b) the development, and (c) the conclusion.
3. The function of the introduction is to attract the reader and that of the conclusion is to leave the reader with your intended message. The function of the development is to encourage the reader to get from opening to conclusion. To do this it must be simple, balanced and logical.

7   Effective Writing

'The hallmark of any great prose is its simplicity', **Ted Bottomley and Anthony Loftus**[18].

If you have followed the steps outlined in the previous chapters, you will now have come to the easiest, or least difficult, stage: the writing. You will have chosen your idea, pinpointed your market and audience, completed your research and drawn up your structure. Now all you have to do is find the right words. This puts in perspective the problem that all writers talk about when they should be writing – the fear of sitting down and staring at a blank piece of paper, or writer's block. You should be bursting to start.

Unfortunately, what should be the easiest and most enjoyable part of the process is often the part that makes good thought unintelligible. Many people, faced with putting their thoughts on paper, adopt a new, and usually unattractive, personality. Most of us can communicate effectively over the dinner table or in our local pub, but once we start writing we are all tempted to use a completely different set of words and constructions. This may come from a conscious desire to impress, or a subconscious regression to schooldays, when teachers gave higher praise for longer words. Whatever the cause, the results are awful.

The aim of this chapter is to help you avoid making sows' ears out of silk purses. The means is style, which is not an excuse to show off but a way of choosing words and putting them together in a way that communicates effectively with your target audience. 'There is no satisfactory explanation of style, no infallible guide to good writing, no assurance that a person who thinks clearly will be able to write clearly, no key that unlocks the door, no inflexible rule by which the young writer may shape his course,' writes E B White[19]. 'He will often find himself steering by stars that are disturbingly in motion.'

It is easier to state what style is not. It is not an excuse to show off your vocabulary or trundle out laboured jokes; personality can and should come through, but it should slide across unobtrusively, reflected subtly in the material you have chosen, the way you have ordered it, and the words you have selected. It does not help the writer to display rococo flourishes, such as using in the first paragraph an obscure word like *ukase* (an edit of Tsarist Russia).

The most effective style for our purpose is that most closely connected with spoken English. Tell a story in a pub and your audience will immediately let you know, with downcast eyes and shuffling feet, when you have lost their interest. They give you instant feedback and you can change your style or content accordingly. Imagine yourself explaining to a typical member of your audience. You will choose the right tone, the right words and constructions, and, as an added bonus, will be guided into the right punctuation.

Bear in mind one principle: *the reader's interests are paramount.* The goal is easily stated: writers must guide the reader from the first word to the last and leave him or her understanding exactly what they mean to say. This is crucial. If it is not done, whatever the writer has to say, however valuable, is worthless. Self-indulgence has destroyed communication.

Writing for the reader is the only absolute rule of this kind of writing. Beware those who tell you otherwise. What follows is a set of guidelines on which most writers on writing agree, but they are guidelines, not rules. You may break them from time to time, but you should do so deliberately, not by default.

Use sentences logically

The principle established in earlier chapters still holds: good writing is rooted in clear thought. This applies to sentences as well as to articles.

Take this example, from a real-life memo: *Following a review of information available from our statistical returns, and a resolution of the last unit care meeting, I would ask you to note that all home visits to customers of our service should be by appointment only.* What happened and when? The passage is confusing because the writer has failed to order the facts, and to use sentences to express them in their proper order. This is, in sequence: (1) the statistical review, (2) the meeting, (3) the resolution and (4) the instruction. Now we know what happened we can plan the sentences logically: *We have carried out a statistical survey of home visits. The last unit care meeting considered the figures and decided that home visits should be by appointment only in future. I would ask you to follow this policy.*

Effective writing is progressive. It is ordered, in time or in some other logical way. Accordingly, sentences should reflect this order; they should not be crammed with ideas. 'The full stop is a great help to sanity,' writes Harold Evans, author of the classic journalism text *Newsman's English* and former editor of *The Sunday Times*[20]. Sentences should also be arranged into paragraphs, each of which makes a coherent point.

Be active, not passive

Another way of blurring a simple message is by using the passive voice. Take this sentence, from the same memo: *It is expected that visits by appointment will be the norm.* But expected by whom? The writer? The committee? Passengers on the 7.15 from Effingham Junction? No-one has been excluded.

Like government forms, the passive seeps everywhere. Democrats hide behind it: notice how rarely committee members decide to raise subscriptions; rather, *It was decided that subscriptions should be raised.* Bureaucrats use it constantly. Take, for example, this sentence from an official circular: *Policies for the control of smoking and the control of alcohol abuse are required not just from the Health Authority but should be extended to the Local Authority as a large employer of labour.* How much better it would have been to have written, in the active: *The Local Authority, as a large employer of labour, should also have policies for the control of smoking and the control of alcohol abuse.* Better still would be *...to control smoking and alcohol abuse...*, but that's another part of this story.

Doctors have taken the passive to their collective heart. Scientific papers are full of equivocal phrases such as *It was observed that...* and *It was discovered that...* . But by whom exactly? Some argue (not, please note: *It is argued...*) that this convention gives a sense of dignity and objectivity, while others counter that it is really a device to make science and scientists appear more important than they really are. Whatever the reason, the habit has now spread to much doctors' writing. It can go to extreme lengths: *It was decided that we should take our holidays in France this year.* (By the district general manager, perhaps?).

The most effective construction in the English language is: subject – (transitive) verb – object. *Jim hits John* gives a precise and economical account. It leaves the reader with no room for doubt. But turn it into the passive – *John was hit by Jim* – and two things happen.

Economy is the first casualty. The active version is short: two words shorter, which for those who like statistical devices, gives an 'AVII' (Albert Verbal Inflation Index) of 66.6 per cent recurring. The passive voice always uses more words: *It was prescribed by his physician* is a wasteful six compared with three for *His physician prescribed. My first night on call will always be remembered by me* can go down from 11 words to 9: *I will always remember my first night on call.*

The second casualty is clearness. This is particularly obvious in phrases such as *It is expected*, but even with the relatively unambiguous action of Jim hitting John, using the passive brings doubt. John may have been hit by Jim, but was it deliberate, or accidental? Whenever you come across the *by* word, as in *It is believed by the Health Department...*, ask yourself who is doing what to whom? In this case the idea is much more simply put by saying *The Health Department believes.* Sometimes the writer will not have made the subject clear, in which case a sub-editor will have to find that out for him or herself, or import one of those useful generic words like *observers, critics, administrators, patients* or *doctors.*

There is a place for the passive. If Jim is languishing in prison on a charge of grievous bodily harm, then he will value the distinction between *John was hit by a brick* and *Jim dropped a brick on John's head.* Also, if John happens to be the Prime Minister of England, then it would be appropriate to start the sentence with him as the subject. But these are exceptions.

Be positive, not negative

Another aid to more vigorous writing is the positive. Many writers tend to tie themselves into *nots*, such as this writer in a learned journal: *Fewer than one junior hospital doctor in 25 would not be prepared to take some form of action in support of shorter working hours.* It is difficult to understand in one reading. Instead turn it into the active: *More than 24 junior hospital doctors out of 25 are prepared to take some form of action in support of shorter working hours.*

'Sentences should assert', writes Harold Evans. 'The ... reader does not want to be told what is not. He should be told what is[20]'. Classic examples include *not often on time* (usually late), *did not remember* (forgot), *not difficult* (easy) and *does not succeed* (fails). The double negative is more than twice as bad: *The lengths of the two lists of candidates were not dissimilar* is much easier to understand when recast as *The two lists of candidates were similar.*

This is not to say that you should not use *not.* But you should not overuse it. Keep it for denial or antithesis, not to mask woolly thinking or as a sop to someone who might be offended. Similarly, save tentative words like *would* and *could* for occasions of real doubt. Writing that fails to assert will leave the reader cold, or at best lukewarm.

Make every word count

Words are the building blocks of writing; they give it meaning and atmosphere and therefore must be chosen with care. The vastness of the English language makes for a formidable landscape, but it can also drag the unwary into a confusion of what Sir Ernest Gowers called 'a small vocabulary of shapeless bundles of uncertain content'[21], words like *position, situation, in terms of*, and *factor*. Like a good night out, words should be specific, simple, suitable and sensuous. The following guidelines should help. They are based on common sense rather than on rules of grammar that most of us have forgotten.

Specific

Vagueness is a major obstacle to effective writing. To quote Harold Evans again: 'A spade should be a spade and not a factor of production. Abstract words should be chased out in favour of specific, concrete words. Sentences should be full of bricks, beds, houses, cars, cows, men and women. Detail should drive out generality. And everything should be related to human beings.[20]' We can go further: even these concrete words can be made more concrete still. Cars can be Fords, Toyotas, Rolls Royces or Ladas. They can be convertibles, hatchbacks, sports cars, or estate wagons. Cows can be Fresians or Jerseys. The more specific you can be, the more vivid the picture. There is no excuse for *termination of life*, as I once read; circumlocution does not take the sting out of death.

Vigorous writing comes from verbs and nouns, not adjectives. Some teachers suggest writing a description of *The best day of my life* – and then cutting out 80 per cent of the adjectives. Words like *pretty* and *old* are vague and dull, and add little. We might be tempted to write *The old man sat outside the pretty cottage, despite the bad weather*, but substitute more concrete words and it is transformed: *The 93-year old former tax-collector sat in the lily pond, while behind him the snow piled up on the slates of his stone cottage.* Each word is simple, but bringing them together builds up an intriguing picture.

Obituaries are full of vague words: *staunch supporter...practical and caring physician...devoted family man...unfailing kindness and devotion to work.* Such phrases are tired words, commonly called clichés (see Figure 7.1), and they make sorry monuments. Avoid stale expressions and seek out concrete words and your writing will be transformed into something original, informal and lively.

Figure 7.1 Avoid like the plague

acid test	add insult to injury
at this point in time	bewildering variety
burning issue	conspicuous by its absence
catalyst for change	cornerstone
draw the line	eminently qualified
frame of reference	foregone conclusion
give the green light	goes without saying
heartfelt thanks	horns of a dilemma
inextricably linked	in the last analysis
monotonous regularity	pillar of the establishment
pros and cons	raise the question
rectify the situation	state of the art
sweeping changes	thin end of the wedge
winds of change	writing on the wall

Not everyone agrees. I was once challenged with an ingenious argument: if we should write as we speak, and, because we often speak in clichés, then good writing should consist of as many clichés as possible. There are two lines of defence. The first is that it is easier to get away with these phrases when we are speaking, and the second is that we probably get away with them far less often than we think. If you know any amateur mimics, you will know that they seize upon stock phrases as much as they do on mannerisms.

You should also make sure that you use the right word. Mrs Malaprop was rightly ridiculed. But there is an important difference between *continuous* and *continual* and good writers will continue to honour it. Of course, language is constantly developing, which is why the use of *partially* (strictly speaking: 'biased', the opposite of 'impartially') is now used instead of *partly*, as witness a recent BBC commentary which talked about 'partially submerged rocks'. (But I still believe that *partially deaf* really means someone who chooses to hear certain things rather than someone who can only hear certain things.) If in doubt, use a dictionary; meanwhile the list in Figure 7.2 may help.

Figure 7.2 Perilous pairs

affect, to influence	**effect**, to accomplish
alternate, succeeding each other	**alternative**, mutually exclusive
appraise, estimate	**apprise**, inform
compare to, liken A to B	**compare with**, note resemblance/ difference
complement, that which completes	**compliment**, expression of praise
continuous, uninterrupted	**continual**, very frequent
deficient, incomplete	**defective**, faulty
defuse, take heat out of	**diffuse**, spread out
dependant, somebody dependent on	**dependent**, depending on
discreet, prudent	**discrete**, separate
disinterested, not biased	**uninterested**, not interested
ensure, to make safe	**insure**, make sure of compensation
explicit, stated in detail	**implicit**, implied
everyone, all	**every one**, each
flaunt, display	**flout**, express contempt for
fortuitous, by chance	**fortunate**, lucky
illusive, deceptive	**elusive**, slippery
infer, deduce	**imply**, hint
ingenious, clever	**ingenuous**, open
militate, tell against	**mitigate**, appease
nauseous, causing sickness	**nauseated**, feeling sick
partial, biased	**in part**, to some degree
stationary, still	**stationery**, writing material
principal, main (person)	**principle**, rule
tortuous, full of turns	**torturous**, inflicting pain
urban, connected with a town	**urbane**, suave

That, defines, as in *the bed that was broken* (ie, the only one that was broken) *has been filled*;
Which, not restrictive, as in *the bed, which was* (ie, happened to be) *broken, has been filled.*

Fewer than/ more than, refer to numbers: *fewer than 120*.
Less than/ over, refer to degree or quantity: *over 17 per cent.*

Simple

Why do we all persist in using a long word when a short one will do just as well? Yet, despite the actions of organizations like the Plain English Campaign, we tend, when writing, to revert to a complicated vocabulary and churn out long words. It is like the default mode on a computer: lose our concentration and sloppy habits appear. Government departments, insurance companies and lawyers are particularly bad; doctors are not immune. Experts say that we should opt for the words derived from

Anglo-Saxon rather than Latin, which isn't a great deal of help if you don't know which is which. Figure 7.3 shows a list of common pomposities; I would not go so far as to say that you should strike them out whenever you see them, but at least ask if they are really necessary.

Figure 7.3 Pomposities

Avoid...	Prefer...	Avoid...	Prefer...
absence of	no	at intervals of	every
additional	more	affect in a positive way	benefit
alternative	other	apparent	clear
approximately	about	assistance	help
attempt	try	at this point in time	now
commencement	start	compared with	than
consequently	so	considerable proportion	many
demonstrate	show	document	report
due to the fact that	because	elevated	higher
fatality	death	females	women
general public	people	in addition	also
in close proximity to	near	in relation to	about
in the course of	during	it is possible that	could
magnitude	size	medical profession	doctors
not only...but also	...and also...	on behalf of	for
participate	take part	performed	did
prior to	before	possesses	has
purchase	buy	reached a conclusion	concluded
regarding	about	remuneration	pay
request	ask	residence	home
retain	keep	reveal	show
shortly	soon	stated	said
substantial number	many	terminate	end
utilization	use	whether	if

Some teachers have gone so far as to develop a 'fog index', which analyses the difficulty of any piece of writing. Take a passage of about 100 words, ending in a full stop. Work out the average sentence length (100 divided by the number of sentences). Then work out the percentage of difficult words, that is, those with three syllables or more. However, ignore two syllable words which have become three syllables with plurals or with endings like -*ed* or -*ing*, technical words (but not jargon) and proper nouns (*Manchester, Winchester*). Add the average sentence length to the number of difficult words and multiply by 0.4 (for example, see Figure 7.4). The result will be the reading score.

Do not confuse this with chronological age: a reading score of 14 and above is believed to be undergraduate standard. It can be a useful test to apply, though it can bring a nasty shock. A survey of practice leaflets showed that their reading score varied from eight to 17, with an average of 11.6. This compared with a reading age of seven for Arthur Hailey, 11 for Kingsley Amis, 16 for a BMJ article on medical audit and 20 for an insurance policy[21].

Figure 7.4 Fog index

Example one
An action group was formed within the *community* by the more *vociferous individuals* in 1989, which included local *councillors*, with the expressed object of campaigning for a local *surgery*. Following a *variety* of *incongruous* and *inconsequential* moves, the group *eventually* approached the *medical* practices whose current *responsibilities* included the village of Dudgeham.

Inexplicably the Patients Action Group did not *communicate* with the *committee* and, therefore, the latter was not afforded the *opportunity* to explain the *parameters* of *provision* for a *surgery* for GMPs nor the limited powers at their *disposal* for *negatively* controlling the *distribution* of *medical* manpower within any given *geographical locality*. (*100 words – three sentences.*)

Example two
Local *councillors* and others formed an action group to campaign for a local *surgery*. They *eventually* approached the doctors who covered the village. The Patients Action Group did not speak to the FHSA, which therefore could not explain the rules for providing a GP *surgery* or its limited powers of controlling where GPs work.

In September 1989 Dr Prodder asked if his practice could open a branch *surgery* in Dudgeham. Our practice premises *manager* inspected the proposed site and decided that, with some *internal* changes, it would be *suitable*. The FHSA gave outline *approval*. (93 words – six sentences.)

	Example one	Example two
Sentence length	33	17
No. of long words	24	9
Total	57	26
Reading score	22.8	10.4

Some argue that long words show education and that short words are degrading and childish. That misses the point. The purpose of writing is to convey information and ideas. Language is the means of doing it, and there is no reason why the process should be over-complicated. If you doubt whether simple language can cope with complex ideas, just consider this statement: 'I think therefore I am'.

Finally, avoid the habit of adding an extra word, either by an extra noun, as in *redundancy situation*; preposition, as in *moving on*: or adjective, as in *lonely hermit*. Again, examples abound (see Figure 7.5). My pet hate is the use of *-wise*, as in *health-wise, money-wise*. This practice has been destroyed by the story of the proud mother owl who said that her baby owl was doing well wise-wise.

Figure 7.5 Redundancy situations

absolute **perfection**	acute **crisis**
best ever	collaborative **link**
completely **unique**	**continue** to remain
dates back from	**during** the course of
entirely **absent**	fairly **unique**
few in number	final **settlement**
general **public**	**he** is a man **who**
interpersonal **relationships**	in the process of **researching**
in two years time	**it is interesting** to note that
major **breakthrough**	**may** possibly
nearly **inevitable**	new **beginning**
oral **contraceptive pill**	period of **one week**
revert back	skin **rashes**
small in size	**smile** on his face
true **facts**	**worst** ever

Suitable

Like all good rules, the rule about short words has its exceptions. These come from a second principle, which is that words should suit the audience and the channel of communication. *Beak raps top doc* uses the shortest words possible. It would do well in the *Sun*, but for a medical paper it would be better to say *Magistrate warns BMA President*. In other words the language must suit the reader, the subject matter and the channel of communication. It would be wrong to say a football game *commenced*, though the word could be used ironically to describe the deliberations (not talks) of a group of medical politicians. However, these are exceptions. Bad writers will let themselves be seduced by long words, but good writers will seek out the most economical. Their goal is to ease the reader's path, not litter it with extravagances.

As already written, professionals writing for lay audiences should take care to avoid jargon. Instead of *establishing the efficacy of this approach* why not *find out if the approach worked*? To take another example: *A prospective study was started using a computer data base; all 427 patients admitted to the unit were examined* becomes *We started a prospective study by using computer data to study all 427 patients admitted to the unit*. The second version is much easier to understand and, if you are in the business of conveying information, this is what you should aim for.

Sensuous

Another exceptional circumstance in which a longer word may be substituted for a shorter one is when the longer word sounds better. In Chapter One, I used the phrase *immersed in bits of paper* rather than *flooded*, having persuaded myself that it conveyed more effectively the depressing nature of it all. This is not an excuse for reverting to long words, but a reminder that, in exceptional cases, they are better (*not* preferable).

If you follow these guidelines, your style will emerge. 'A careful and honest writer does not need to worry about style,' writes E B White. 'As he becomes proficient in the use of the language, his style will emerge, because he himself will emerge, and when this happens he will find it increasingly easy to break through the barriers that separate him from other minds, other hearts – which is, of course, the purpose of writing, as well as its principal reward.'[19]

Key points

1. Effective writing takes the reader from beginning to end leaving him with an understanding of exactly what is being said. The reader's interests are paramount.
2. Use sentences logically. Use verbs in the active voice. Use positives rather than negatives. Words should be specific, simple, suitable and sensuous.
3. If you follow these guidelines, your style will emerge.

8   Revision

'To forge simple direct prose you need to rewrite and rewrite and rewrite and rewrite', **Michael O'Donnell**[23].

So now the great work is finished. You can print it (or take it out of your typewriter), put it in an envelope, and address it to the editor. You can wallow with satisfaction in a job well done.

Wrong. This was only the first draft. You now have to work on it again, to make sure that it really fulfils the brief you set yourself. The first stage is to leave it, at least overnight and preferably a week, and then come back to it. It will look sadly tarnished.

This is the time for fine tuning, and occasionally for starting afresh. Revision is not an activity to be tacked on to your writing, but an integral stage – the fifth and last – whose importance can never be overstated. Most writers do it, and good writers spend longer at it than most. Like most things in life, effortlessness takes hard work and practice. If you are on a deadline, make sure you leave time for this part of the process.

Some people say that you should read your article at least twice, looking first at the article as a whole, and then looking at the technical details. The only drawback with this process is that it is a waste of time unless you know which questions to ask. Many of them have already been covered in various parts of this book, but this chapter will bring them together again, and provide a checklist (Figure 8.1). The list of questions may be relatively short; not so the process of asking them.

Structure

Overview

Does your article fulfil your brief? If you are satisfied that it does, put yourself in the eyes of your target reader, and ask again if the brief is worthwhile. Have you made it interesting? Have you proved your thesis?

Can your argument be torn apart? Are there inconsistencies? When you are satisfied, look for more specific structural points.

Figure 8.1 Writing articles: a checklist

Structural:

- Is what I am trying to say clear (ie, can I sum it up in one sentence?)
- Do I grab the reader?
- Is there enough to hold his/ her attention?
- Do I leave him/ her with a clear conclusion?
- Is my structure clear? (An article is made up of argument and illustration, so can the reader skim it?) – Is the argument logical?
- Are quotes used correctly, to illustrate rather than develop the argument?
- Is my attention wavering?
- Is there information which (though interesting) does not add to the argument, and therefore should be in a box or table?
- Does the article have any flaws or omissions?
- How can my argument be criticized?
- Are the steps logical and easy to follow? Or do I repeat myself or make sudden leaps?

Technical:

- Do I have to read anything twice?
- Am I using the active?
- Am I using positives?
- Are the words/ phrases the right ones?
- Are the sentences/ paragraphs too long and complicated?
- Are there any literals or spelling mistakes?
- Are there any major grammatical errors?
- Can I prove my facts?
- Are quotes and the opinions of others clearly attributed?
- Is there any danger of libel?
- Are my opinions clearly justified (and not merely justifiable)?
- Are any phrases cumbersome?
- Is the language pompous, obscure, bureaucratic?
- Will the reader have any unanswered questions?
- Is it in house style?

Introductions

Does the introduction really attract the reader and set up a 'dynamic' that the reader will want to pursue? At this stage you may wish to insert one, for example: *This illustrates the difficulty of finding NHS managers who know anything about patients' needs* or *This is a story of lust and love in British hospitals which demonstrates beyond any manner of doubt that crime really does pay*. Try cutting out the first paragraph to see whether you have succumbed to a bout of throat-clearing. Be brave: however much pain went into a word or phrase, throw it out if it adds nothing to the article as a whole.

Closings

The opening may work, but what about the conclusion? Will you leave the reader with the message that you intended? Have you written a conclusion, or simply come to a halt? Will your conclusion stimulate readers, or will they simply say *So what* and turn to the next page? If you leave the reader with a question, will he or she have enough information to answer it?

Here it is important to distinguish between the deliberate *stimulating* question and the unintended *perplexing* question. With the first, the readers are given enough facts and challenged to make up their own minds; with the second, readers are left unsatisfied because important issues have been hinted at and not resolved. To take an obvious example, writing that this is the *second biggest ... in the world* begs the question: what is the biggest? If you can't answer it without destroying the flow of your article, leave it out. If you can't leave it out, rework your structure so that you can put in the answer. Don't just tack it on.

Development

Now turn to the way you have built up your argument. Will a stranger to the subject, and to you, be able to follow it clearly without having to read it again? Or do you need to make your structure more obvious? Sometimes an extra sentence at the start of a paragraph will do, or even a single word like *However, Nevertheless* or *Meanwhile*. Beware of using quotations to develop the argument because readers tend to read them as illustration and may miss the fact that they contain an important development. Check whether there is a mass of information that would be better off in a box or table.

Good articles are made out of 'bones' and 'flesh'. The 'bones' are the essential parts of the argument and the 'flesh' is the supporting material. Look at the structure by highlighting with a yellow marker pen all those sentences which are essential. If the yellow lines are evenly spaced, the structure will be good. But, if they are unbalanced or concentrated in one part of the article, you may need to rethink.

Finally watch out for your own reactions. If you are getting bored, then what chance has the reader?

Filling in gaps

Some writers find it easier to write the first draft straight through, without referring to the facts they have collected. There is nothing wrong with that; it has the advantage of allowing you to concentrate on getting the structure right. But, if this is how you choose to write, now is the time to fill in the gaps.

Technique

Facts

Watch particularly for names: Robin Smith may sound straightforward, but what about Robyn Smyth? You may develop an instinct for spotting your mistakes, but there is no substitute for checking and re-checking. Nothing devalues an article as much as a fact that is wrong. It could lose you the support of readers and editor, and could mean that you have wasted your work. Use reference books. Use the telephone. Ask yourself constantly: do I really know that this is correct, or am I making an assumption?

Style

Now check the style. Is it easy to understand? Is it self-indulgent? Do you have to read anything twice? Comb your writing to see where you have unwittingly flouted (not flaunted) the guidelines: watch for the *by* words and unravel the *nots*. Delete flights of fancy and weed out clichés, pomposities and jargon. They will almost certainly appear (as did a remarkable number of passives in the first draft of this book, particularly in the section on avoiding the passive).

All good publications have an agreed house style. This can vary from a brief list of general principles to bulky documents trying to cover all eventualities. (See Figure 8.2 for some of the main issues). A few have been published. As the version put out by the *New York Times* says: 'There is little difference between a martini and a Martini, but unless there is a style rule the word may be capitalized in one instance and lower-cased in another. Such untidiness must be avoided, in matters small or large, because it detracts from even the best of writing.'[24]

Figure 8.2 Questions of style

Acronyms: Most common style is to use capitals if each letter is pronounced, otherwise upper and lower case: *BBC*, *WHO* but *Unesco* and (logically if you follow this style, but controversially) *Aids*.
Amongst: Archaic waste of two letters. Prefer *among*. Similarly *while* not *whilst*, *amid* not *amidst*.

Brackets: Keep to a minimum. Dashes look better and are now acceptable.

Capitals: Slow the reader down and should also be kept to a minimum.
Christian names: This term is not appropriate for multiracial societies. Prefer *first name*.
Colons: Used to denote that the following words qualify or explain. *He looked at the leg: it was made of steel and glass.*
Comprise: Does not take of. But *consist of.*

Exclamation marks: Overdone. Should be used (sparingly) for exclamations, and not to signal weak jokes.
Etc: Use when a list is really too long, and not because you can't be bothered to think of any more examples.

Get: Can be used if you really can't find an acceptable alternative.

His: Applies only to male possessions. Unfortunately language has not kept pace with our awareness of sexism. Use *his* or *her*, or put into plural, as in *their*.
Hopefully: Technically wrong when used for *I hope*, as in *Hopefully, the lunch will be good.* (Are the sausages being optimistic?). Some commentators feel that this is now so common (and even used by the headmistress in *Neighbours*) that it is now acceptable.
Hyphens: Use sparingly, when they point the reader to the right meaning, as in *answered carefully-prepared questions* or *answered carefully prepared-questions*.

Include: Splendid word for writers, because it allows for any complaint that the list is incomplete and solves the etc. problem.

Lists: Be consistent: *(1), (2), (3); (a), (b), (c)*, or blobs. See style book of target publication for guidance.

Monologophobia: The fear of using the same word more than once in the same passage. This fear is overrated.

Numbers: One to nine, then 10, 11 etc. Usually 1 per cent, 1 cm etc. Avoid starting a sentence with a number.

Quotation marks: Some publications use double quotation marks, some single. Follow style wherever possible. The argument that single words should take single quotation marks is specious. Slang words rarely need them.

Quotation marks and full stops: If the quotation is only part of the sentence, finish it with the quotation mark before putting the full stop: *He said it was an 'appalling waste of money'.* and *'It is an appalling waste of money.'*

Semi-colons: Longer pause than a comma, shorter than a full stop. Used in sentences where there is a logical link but no conjunction (*and, but*). Beware over-use in lists; commas will usually do.

Shall/ will: Current consensus is that the first person (*I* and *we*) takes shall; the second and third (*you, he, she, they*) takes will. Change to *will* and *shall* for emphasis.

Till: Used to put money into. Not to be confused with *until.*

Trade names: Take capitals: *Elastoplast, Sellotape, Thermos.* Alternatives are sticking plaster, adhesive tape or vacuum flask.

Try: Takes *to* not *and.*

Very: Use very occasionally.

NOTE: These are personal views. Editors will have different ideas, but they should be explained in their style sheets.

Policing this style is the job of sub-editors; writers are not expected to know all the details. But they should know the more obvious ones, such as whether the publication uses *Mr* or *Mr..*

Finally, check for careless use of gender. Have you avoided the trap of making all doctors male and all patients female? This is easy to spot, but hard to rectify. Using *he or she* can become tedious. One of the best tricks is to use the plural, so that instead of *doctor...he...* we have *doctors...they... .*

Grammar

Grammar is overrated. Language is a living thing, and its purpose is not to provide a set of rules to be obeyed at all costs, but to provide a framework which will allow us to be understood. Time is better spent on making sure that your argument is well-structured and your choice of words apposite than it is on hunting out split infinitives. I am delighted that no less an authority than Gowers agrees: 'Too much importance is still attached to grammarians' fetishes and too little to choosing the right words'.[25]

Nevertheless, illiteracy is another thing altogether, and Gowers adds:

Figure 8.3 Common grammatical mistakes

1. **Verbless sentences**: Can be used occasionally for effect, but often creep in through ignorance and faulty punctuation, as in: *There is a high incidence of deaths from coronary heart disease. The high consumption of cigarettes being an important factor.*

2. **Floating commas**: Commas must travel in pairs when used for subordinate clauses. *The administrators, who arrived late took over the meeting* should be *The administrators, who arrived late, opened the meeting,* or (note the difference): *The administrators who arrived late took over the meeting.*

3. **Punctuated possessives**: In general, the apostrophe comes before the *s* for singular (*one doctor's*) and after the *s* for the plural (*several doctors'*). Most people now agree that *'s* can go after *s* (*St James's*), but avoid if unbearably ugly: *The book by Sir Ernest Gowers* rather than *Sir Ernest Gowers's book.*

4. **Wandering apostrophes**: Many people are confused about 'its' and 'it's'. It may break the 'rule' about possessives but is easy to remember: imagine that the apostrophe stands for an *i*: *its life* compared with *it's (it is) life.*

5. **Dangling modifiers**: The habit of qualifying something which is not mentioned until later in the sentence, or not at all. As in *Unable to speak, the doctor gave me an enema* or *The chairman having spoken eloquently, the meeting ended on time.*

6. **Misplaced phrases**: Connected phrases should stay together, and not wander off to the other end of the sentence, as in *We talked about several diseases in the restaurant.*

7. **Tense situations**: Stick to one time-frame and keep to it. Not: *The speaker added...He also says... .*

8. **Singular pluralities**: The subject of a sentence must agree with the verb. *Doctors and nurses has a good time* is obviously wrong, but it gets complicated when collective nouns are introduced: *The group of politicians was...*or *Each of the students has a postgraduate degree.*

9. **Problematic pronouns**: Use *I, he she,* and *we* only if they are the subject of the sentence; otherwise *me, him, her* and *us.* Thus *she and I were arguing with him* and *he was arguing with her and me.*

10. **Subtle subjunctives**: *If, provided that* takes the subjunctive: *If I were minister of health... .*

Figure 8.4 Unsaddled hobby horses

1. **Split infinitives**: Many 'experts' now say that you should be guided by your ear, not by this 'rule'. Sometimes the position of the intruding word can make a difference. Does *fail totally to understand the question* mean the same as *fail to understand totally the question*.

2. **Starting a sentence with 'and' or 'but'**: Gowers (3rd edition) states clearly on page 98 that the idea that this is inelegant is now dead. It is not our place to argue.

3. **Ending with a preposition**: Churchill killed this 'rule' when he said it was an idea 'up with which he would not put.' Again, be guided by your ear.

'We cannot have grammar jettisoned altogether; that would mean chaos'. Too many doctors spoil a good impression by making such elementary mistakes as writing *it's* when they should write *its*. The accompanying list (Figure 8.3) covers some of the most common mistakes.

Literals

Now is also the time to look for spelling mistakes, or literals. Does it say *wee* when you meant to say *week*, or is the relationship *casual* when you really mean *causal*? More seriously, has a *not* crept in or a decimal point moved to the left? Those errors could be libellous, or, in the case of dosages, fatal. Have you had a brainstorm and put in the name of that difficult patient instead of the secretary of a medical trade union? Such mistakes do happen. They are easy to make – after all they are one small action, compared with the whole range of decisions that you have been making – but, unspotted, they will spoil any good impression you might have made.

Computerized spelling checks can help, but do not rely on them completely. Many of them are American by inclination, and none of them can be relied upon to register when a good word is in the 'wrong lace'. As here.

There is no substitute for proofreading, but it is neither easy nor interesting. We tend to read what we expect. Some professional proof-readers suggest that you should read backwards, but this is drastic. What you need is peace and quiet and concentration. You also need to home in on things that matter, by which I mean those that could have serious repercussions.

Figure 8.5 Common spelling mistakes

abscess	accommodation	achievement
ageing*	allotted	argument
attendance	beginning	believe
benefited	committee	consensus
definitely	diagrammatic	diarrhoea*
dissatisfaction	embarrass	excerpts
forty	fulfil	gauge
grey*	guarantee	haemorrhage*
homoeopathy*	humorous	hygienic
immediately	independent	indispensable
innocuous	irresistible	liaison
manoeuvre*	miscellaneous	occurrence
oedema*	omitted	ophthalmology
parallel	perseverance	privilege
referral	resuscitation	rhythm
sieve	successful	tumour*
unnecessary	until	

NOTE: Those marked with * are UK versions and differ in American spelling.

Refereeing

If you have time, pass your article to somebody else to read. Some say that the ideal number is three. The first is your partner, who will pick up, usually with undisguised glee, the wandering comma and the inevitable misprint. (It may do little for your relationship, but that is a minor matter in comparison with getting your name in print.) The second is a typical reader, who will be able to tell you whether the article is comprehensible and interesting. For instance, if you are writing for a GP newspaper, ask a GP; if you are writing for the Health Page of the *Guardian*, seek if you can a friendly *Guardian* reader. Finally, show your article to someone who knows the subject well: he or she should be able to spot the major errors.

Journalists are taught that they should never show their article to their subject. I have mixed feelings about that. It can lead to your softening the tone, not necessarily consciously. But non-professional journalists might do well to go back to their source: these will tend to be too picky, and insist on nuances which might reflect them in a better light, but they will almost certainly spot one or two errors of fact. It is a trade-off that can be useful. If you decide to do it, make it clear that you have the last word. The writer should be in control, though this can be difficult if you are a senior house officer and your source is a consultant.

Legal issues

Now is the time to check whether your article is likely to run into legal difficulties. The two major problems are likely to be copyright and defamation.

Copyright

Copyright laws exist to protect against plagiarism. In other words, you must not take a substantial part of someone else's work and present it as your own. There is nothing wrong with quoting what someone has written or said – *provided that you attribute it clearly to the original author*. If you use more than 100 words or so, then you should seek permission from the publisher; it is usually given, without charge. Most writers agree that these rules are sensible enough; after all, they are there to protect them.

Defamation

The laws of defamation are more serious. The time it takes for lawyers to settle an alleged libel can be as long as it takes to settle a case of medical negligence, and, if you are taken to court, the penalties can be just as high and, with our jury system, just as variable. In essence, defamation means that you have harmed somebody's reputation, or, to quote some of the legal phrases, 'exposed them to hatred, ridicule or contempt' or 'lowered them in the estimation of right-thinking members of society generally.' This can sometimes be a subtle distinction: in a review, for example, you may say that the author has written a bad book because we can all write bad books, but saying that he is an incompetent writer or bad scientist could be defamatory.

There are two types of defamation: slander, which is spoken, and libel, which is written. All those concerned with the publication of a libel can be held responsible: editor, publisher and printer as well as writer. Usually the first solicitor's letter will go to your editor, but, if you do ever receive one, the first thing to do is to contact your commissioning editor. Most publications have libel insurance and legal advisers, and they will usually take up the case for, or with you. On no account try to deal with a libel yourself because you could well make matters worse.

If the matter is taken up, you will have three defences. The first is that what you have said is true; in other words everything is factual and you have enough evidence to take to court to prove it. The second is that it is fair comment; in other words these are opinions honestly held. The third defence is privilege; this means that the proceedings of some bodies, such as parliament or the courts, are totally covered, and anything that is said in them can be reported without fear of libel. This explains why, from time to time, Members of Parliament challenge colleagues to come outside and repeat what they have just said. This is not so that they can be beaten up, but because their allegations, once repeated outside, will no longer be covered by privilege.

However, the existence of these defences will not necessarily stop anyone from proceeding with a case, and therefore the prudent writer will avoid defamation wherever possible. The simple rule is not to write anything that puts another person in a bad light, even if you are quoting somebody else. This can often be done accidentally, for example praising a medical politician for spending all his time at committee meetings could imply that he is a lousy doctor. If you want to attack someone who you believe has done wrong, then the laws don't forbid you; they try to ensure that you have good reason for doing so. If you want to go down this line, then talk to your commissioning editor.

Key points

1. Writing does not finish with the last word. Good writers will revise. And revise again... .
2. Look first to see whether the article has any major flaws of design or argument. Then look for technical faults, such as grammatical and typographical errors.
3. Do not take other people's work and present it as your own. Be careful about writing anything that is likely to injure another's reputation.

9   Selling your Article

'Editors are easily pleased, but not often', **Alistair Brewis**[26].

You now have your product. All that remains is to package it so that it has the greatest chance of being published. In other words, you must market this precious piece of your soul.

If you find the use of the *m-* word offensive, swallow your pride in the interests of publication. Put yourself in the position of the person who is about to receive your article. They may know nothing about you, in which case they will have to judge on the evidence available. If they can spot a major error of fact, and they will be looking for one, they will think you unreliable. If they think that your presentation is sloppy, they will be tempted to think that your research has been sloppy. Even if you are a well-established writer, don't take things for granted: editors think they are doing their job when they turn something down, and the bigger the name the better they think they are doing.

Submission

Strategy

Submit only one article at a time. Editors may lose sleep at the prospect of empty pages, but they are incurable optimists. They believe that a better piece will come with every postbag, and so will not commit themselves and their budget to a number of articles from one writer at one time. Also, sending off a pile of articles can give a bad impression: why has this writer written so much and sold so little?

New writers sometimes write to editors suggesting that they should be invited to write a regular column after the enclosed is published. This is presumptuous. Columns are extremely difficult to sustain, and therefore entrusted only to those who have proved themselves over a reasonable length of time. No editor will think of offering one on the basis of one article. If you harbour such ambitions, keep them to yourself for the time being.

Tactics

Make sure that the article is neatly typed, not handwritten. Remember that editors have full timetables and constant deadlines, and resent having to spend time deciphering the undecipherable. They may make time to read it, but you will have started with a disadvantage.

Make sure that your article is double-spaced: this is not just for cosmetic reasons but because changes cannot easily be made on single-spaced manuscripts, and you should not be seen to presume that your article will not need any sub-editing. Put your name, the name of the publication and the date on the top left hand corner. On the top right hand corner put a 'catch line': this is a short label of two syllables, at most, which will be numbered consecutively and which will enable your editor to reassemble the whole when the staple comes out (see Figure 9.1). For the same reason, write *more* or *mf* (more follows) at the bottom of each page, and *ends* at the end. If you can, end each page with a complete paragraph, which also makes it easier for sub-editors.

Headings

Headings give new writers considerable heartache. They may spend hours honing them, be extremely proud of them and then complain when they do not appear. One reason is that they tend to write a *title*, a label which the writer often feels is extremely witty, or sums up his or her feelings about the work. Editors will want a *headline*, which is a stronger and longer statement, usually with a verb and as many emotive words as possible, and aimed at persuading the reader that the article is worth reading. There is another reason: sub-editors write the headline at the last moment, when the page has been designed, and therefore the number of characters will be strictly defined. Writers will be extremely lucky if their version actually fits.

This does not mean that writers should not put a heading on their work. But its function should be to help market the article to an editor. It will rarely appear in the published version.

Covering letters

With your well-presented article you should also send a brief covering letter. Address it to the editor by name; looking in the magazine or making a quick telephone call to the switchboard should give you the information you need, but make sure you get the spelling right. In your letter you will need to establish three things. The first is who you are. This does not mean that you have to send a full CV, but it will help an editor to place you if you write it on official notepaper, with your qualifications mentioned but not flaunted. These should only concern the bits of your life that answer the questions: *Is this person qualified to write on this subject?* and *Is he or she likely to be reliable?*

Second, an editor will also want to know what the article is about. You should have no trouble with this if you have formulated a brief, and kept to it. Again, keep it short and to the point.

Figure 9.1 Sample letter

from Dr JDR Macclesfield, MD MB BS FRCPsych   **St Kenneth's Hospital**
Waldegrave Street
London

John Smith
The Editor
Medical Express
Wapping.

Dear Mr Smith,

I enclose an article on the medical dangers of freelance writing which might suit your Talking Point section. It argues that this hobby, which more and more people are taking up, could result in serious psychiatric disorders. Proper treatment could save the NHS £1.2 million a year.

I have been a consultant psychiatrist at this hospital for 17 years and have treated several cases of severely depressed writers in that time. I have also written three plays, a novel and a slim volume of verse.

I look forward to hearing from you.

Yours sincerely

James Macclesfield

Third, use a sentence (or two at most) to say why you think the readers will be interested at this time. Do not tell the editor what to do: *I think you should publish this immediately because...* is the equivalent of a patient offering his own diagnosis. Instead, give the necessary information in a non-threatening way: *This is a talking point at the moment because....* Don't preface your remarks by saying that you don't value the publication anyway (Yes, it does happen). Editors are as sensitive as other people, and as vindictive.

If the publication asks for a stamped addressed envelope then you should send one. But many publications are gracious enough to spend the few pence on postage.

Don't exceed your skills, for example by offering to draw a sketch or take some photographs. Most publications employ highly skilled and expensive people to do this and will look upon the suggestion as amateur. You can make an exception to this if you have some snaps of a far-away place or a one-off incident, in which case the rarity value may counterbalance the lack of quality.

Finally, make sure you leave a telephone number, and that you can be contacted on it, during the day when *they* are at work.

Figure 9.2 Presenting an article

John Smith/ Medical Telegraph/ June 1993   Writing – 1

Too many doctors are learning how to write. That was the theme of a conference held at the Queen Anne Conference Centre at Withington last week.

Dr Michael Chertsey from Dunstable argued that introducing English into the undergraduate medical curriculum had brought about a new generation. Young doctors were now able to contribute to the journals without being radically rewritten.

'This is a total disgrace,' he said. 'My generation was never taught fringe things like learning to write. We did that at school.

'Now youngsters are coming along who have been spoon-fed with simple words. They even read books in their spare time.

'It is time that this nonsense stopped.'

The long wait

What happens next? In most cases there will be a resounding silence. This is extremely frustrating for writers, whose days and nights will be spent agonizing over the fate of their masterpiece. For the editor, on the other hand, this article will be one of many.

They use 'triage'. All articles are logged in. Some are so terrible that they can be sent back almost immediately. A tiny minority are so good that they can be accepted just as quickly. Most of them will be borderline, and so will be circulated around the staff for second, third and fourth opinions. They may even be put into in-trays which effectively put off the need to take any decision, sometimes for ever.

If you haven't heard anything for a few weeks, then you can make a telephone call. Don't demand to speak to the editor but speak to the secretary and explain that you have heard nothing. You may be able to blame the Post Office. Secretaries will rarely be able to give you an immediate answer, but they should ring you back with a progress report.

Rejection

Don't be surprised if your article is rejected. This happens to everybody at one time or another, and you should try to be positive. You should face the fact that you have failed, but this is not the same as saying that you are a failure (see section on libel). It may not be your fault: perhaps the editor had already asked someone else to write on the same subject. On the other hand, if you have made mistakes, you should try to find out what they were.

The rejection letter may not give you an answer. Editors tend to hide behind anodyne phrases, such as *I much enjoyed reading your article but I'm afraid we haven't got space at the present time.* That doesn't mean to say that you shouldn't ask for the editor's opinion, but be careful: it is as hard to give criticism as it is to take it. It also takes a lot of time. Some editors won't thank me for saying this, but there is nothing wrong in phoning back and asking for some pointers. But be tactful, and, when or if they come, be humble and listen: on no account start arguing.

You should also look for another market. One of the good things about the British press is that editors vary in their opinions, and what one may reject another may seize gratefully. They won't be offended if they see an article they have rejected turning up somewhere else; in fact it will reinforce their belief that their publication has higher standards. Keep trying, though make sure that you only send to one at a time, and that you remember to change the name of the publication on the top of the first page.

Acceptance

You may, on the other hand, have received an acceptance letter. Savour the moment, then remind yourself that there are still pitfalls ahead.

Dealing with sub-editors

While you are working out your acceptance speech for the Nobel Prize for Literature, your article will be making its way from editor to sub-editors. Their job is to turn such raw material into the form that they think their readers will most readily accept and this ranges from a slight polish to a structural upheaval, or 'scissors and paste' job. This process is sensitive. Authors understandably feel threatened when their precious phrasing is altered. Sub-editors understandably feel threatened when their hard work is met by wounded pride: they see themselves as hard-worked casualty officers routinely reviving corpses, only to be met with complaints that some of the patient's jacket buttons are now missing.

Proofs

Some publications send the author a proof of the sub-edited work. They are taking a risk. They know that this will help to reduce errors, but it can be time-consuming and ego-threatening. Don't be discouraged when you see the changes: again, consider why they were made. You may think that the sub-editors have destroyed your personality, but were they doing you a favour? You may think that they have misunderstood the points you were trying to make, but did you make them clearly in the first place?

You can smooth this part of the process in two ways. First, send back your corrections by the given deadline. If they are too late the sub-editor has two alternatives: ignore them, or go through the expensive process of asking the printers to make the page again. Neither are satisfactory. Second, make as few comments as possible, and limit these to questions of accuracy, not style.

If you are really unhappy with the result, and feel that it now seriously misrepresents your opinions, then you should mention this to the sub-editor. Try not to personalize it, and on no account threaten to go over his or her head to the editor. If you remain unhappy, ask the sub-editor to speak to the editor about it, and to call you back. These are drastic measures; the chances of your original version being reinstated are slim. The best you can hope for is that the article is taken out or your name removed. Both options will inconvenience the editorial staff, and you may well find (as I did on the only occasion that I felt I had to ask for my name to be removed) that you are quietly dropped as a contributor.

Publication

The next stage should be seeing your article in print. Once you have got over the thrill of seeing your name in biggish letters, and if you haven't already seen a proof, you will start to notice that changes have been made. The same principle applies: cause trouble only if you feel you must. The options are to telephone the editor to put your point of view, or write a letter for publication. Again, be aware that this might ruin a promising partnership.

On the other hand, you may find that your article, though accepted, still does not appear. When can you start chasing it up? Leave it for several issues. The editor may well have changed his or her mind, but more probably the piece has been overtaken by more timely articles. You can make a polite call to the editor, or, better still, the editorial assistant. Don't be aggressive (*You have had this article for weeks and NOTHING HAS BEEN DONE...*), but ask politely for a progress report (*Do you have any news as to when it might be published?*).

The editor might give you a date, or say that they no longer wish to use it and offer to send it back. Those situations are straightforward. A third option is that they have not yet scheduled it, but still want to hang on to it. You have the right to ask for it back, though not be paid. It's probably better to let them keep it a little while longer.

Payment

Money can often ruin a promising relationship. Within two months of publication you should receive a cheque. It will probably be based on standard rates, and unlikely to be a great amount. Accept it gratefully. It is tactless to complain to journalists that you are badly paid; they will almost certainly be earning much less money than you.

Once you are an established writer, you should try to establish before each commission how much you will be paid. Good publications will send you a letter confirming this point; if they do not, you can always write a confirmatory letter yourself. Try to appear businesslike, not greedy.

Figure 9.3 Do's and don'ts of dealing with editors

DO:
- target properly
- present well
- be considerate
- be helpful
- put your name on copy
- keep a spare
- keep to deadlines.

DON'T:
- be too clever
- be a nuisance
- be wrong
- argue unnecessarily
- be petty about money
- submit more than one article
- send to more than one editor at a time.

Key points

1. Market your product to the editor. This means presenting a clear typescript and sending a brief covering letter.
2. Rejections are inevitable: profit from them by trying to work out where you went wrong. Don't be afraid to revise your article and send it elsewhere.
3. If your article is accepted, make sure that you deal sensitively with staff throughout the process of sub-editing.

10   Where Do We Go From Here?

'The world of medical journalism is small, varied, and bitchy and is probably not for the faint hearted, but may be an endless source of amusement to the thick-skinned divergent thinker', **Stella Lowry and Richard Smith**[27].

Welcome to the world of writers. Almost.

By now you should have had your first article published. But, as Lady Bracknell might have said, doing something once is an accident, but doing it twice demands talent. Repeating an initial success can be difficult, though it can get easier thereafter. Take stock of your situation, and ask: do you want to go through all that again? If so, where do you want to end up?

Look back at the strategy you set yourself. If you intended to write only one article, read no further. But if you find that you are becoming addicted, you will almost certainly have to extend into other markets and try other types of writing. You may also wish to improve your skills, or even take up writing as a full-time career. This chapter aims to explore these urges.

Building up relationships

One of the delights of writing, which almost compensates for those dull days where words fail and articles get rejected, is the unexpected commission. Imagine the scene: you are sitting alone depressed, with not an idea in sight. Suddenly the phone rings. A commissioning editor wants you to go to Honolulu to report a conference, with all expenses paid plus generous fees. Or write 500 words before breakfast on the latest study on circulatory disorders.

Whatever the subject, such phone calls are good for a writer's delicate ego. They also provide a welcome challenge by forcing us, with pay, to analyse and report issues to which we have probably never given much thought. One person has a limited number of ideas, so being handed other people's increases our range. The long-term aim should be to position yourself so that commissioning editors are constantly ringing you up. This is difficult.

Building on your contacts

Build on the contact you have already made. Provided that your article was acceptable, and that the production process went smoothly, you should now be established as a good and reliable writer. This is important; you are no longer marketing a single article but yourself as a writer.

Submit something else. Timing is important: too long an interval and you will be forgotten; too short and you will risk appearing desperate. Now they know what you can do, you can submit an idea rather than a finished article. This can be tricky: if you only give one you could be left with a straight rejection, and, if you give too many, it looks as if you lack confidence. Three or four is probably a good number, but there can be no rigid guide.

If you choose to submit one idea, put it in a letter; if you choose to send more than one, write a covering letter with your ideas on a separate sheet. Remind them about the article they have published. Try a bit of flattery or a thank you, but don't grovel. Give the idea simply – the chapter on writing the brief should help you do this – with some idea of how you propose to get the material. Put it in context: why will it interest the readers? Why is it topical? Why should *you* do it?

What happens if your idea is rejected, and later turns up in the same publication? You have two choices. You can take the charitable view that, large organizations being what they are, the idea has bubbled up quite innocently from another quarter, and say nothing. Or you can assume that someone has ripped you off and protest. This is unlikely to have any useful result.

After a while you can start dealing by phone. This is easier than writing, because you will get an instant reaction, and the opportunity to trim your offering accordingly. One day the editor may invite you to lunch, and, if so, take one or two good ideas with you. You should not try to sell them immediately: the editor may well have an idea for you, or you may hit upon a new idea together.

Good reputations circulate round offices, though not so fast as bad ones. You may have written a feature article on your experience of Voluntary Service Overseas. The books editor may see it and ask you to review a book on medicine in the third world. The news editor may ask you to cover a conference on *Stepping off the career ladder*. And so on. For this to work, you need to have a reputation for reliability, you need to be fresh in their memories, and you need to have a certain amount of luck.

Breaking into new publications

The best way of expanding your contacts is to start the process all over again, from brief to submission. Now, however, you will be a published author, which should bring confidence and, more important, a cutting you can send as proof of competence. All editors are reassured by the fact that a colleague has backed you into print.

Another way of extending your contacts comes from the fact that journalists keep changing jobs. This is good news. Make sure that, whenever your commissioning editor moves on, you know where they are going. Ask them to introduce you to their successor and you will now have two contacts.

Sometimes the chemistry between you and the new editor will be wrong, with no fault attached to either side. Sometimes he or she will want to change in a way which you feel you cannot, or do not want, to follow. Sometimes they will bring in new writers. Don't be depressed: for every editor who thinks your work is bad, there is probably another who thinks it is terrific.

Syndication and recycling

Research often provides far too much information for each story. At the conference on *Stepping Off the Career Ladder*, for instance, did a speaker give details of an interesting line of research that could be expanded into an interesting article? Was there a paper by a doctor who now runs a windsurfing academy, which could be worked into another article, perhaps for a general interest paper? Did a member of the audience make a controversial point that could provide the theme for an opinion piece? It is a good exercise to write down two or three follow-ups. You can offer some to the same publication, in which case they will be impressed by your eagerness, or you can try other markets.

Editors will have every right to be aggrieved if you submit a similar article to a competitor, but you should have no trouble if you wish to reshape your article for another audience. Some nurses may have spoken to the conference, in which case you could use their contributions for an article in the nursing press. Editors should not object to this, though out of courtesy you should tell them, particularly if they paid your expenses for the conference in the first place.

If you want to make as much money as possible for no extra effort, syndicate your article, in other words sell it as it is to another publication. Here you must beware of copyright. Under the 1988 Copyright Designs and Patents Act, all authors own their own articles. However, many publications, particularly those with active syndication departments, now insist that you sign these away when your article is accepted. Whether they have the right to do this is not the point: once again it is a question of whether the effort and cost of resisting is worthwhile, particularly at the start of a writing career. If you see a real opportunity for repeat sales, try to persuade them to accept First British Rights only. But consider an informal approach first; most editors will act fairly.

Getting an agent

A common question from tyro writers is: *Should I have an agent?* The simplest answer is: *Not yet.*

The main reason for having an agent is not to frighten a commissioning editor, though it may well do, but to negotiate on your behalf. It follows that you must have something worth negotiating. In general, most writers for newspapers and magazines will use their own contacts and negotiate their own rates. Some authors will do so for textbooks and other non-fiction works, thus saving the 10 or 15 per cent commission. But where an agent will come into his or her own is for a book, probably a novel, which has possibilities for spin-offs, such as TV or radio rights, or where the writer does not want to bother negotiating with a number of publishers. Another advantage is that, if a good agent agrees to represent you, he or she should be able to advise on the best way to proceed with your work.

To find an agent look in a reference book like the *Writer's and Artist's Yearbook* or the *Writer's Handbook*. Your approach to an agent will differ little from an approach to a commissioning editor. Agents will want to know whether you have a product worth spending their time on, so send a polite covering letter with an outline or synopsis of the proposed work and a sample of your work. Do not delude yourself that they will be falling over themselves to represent you: they only take on a small proportion of people who approach them. If you want your work returned, enclose a stamped addressed envelope.

Finally, you would do well to remember Michael O'Donnell's advice: 'However brazen your agent, only you can earn the money'[28].

Professionalism

To succeed in the harsh world of freelance writing you will need to build up a certain amount of what is nowadays called professionalism, but what old fashioned hacks such as myself like to think of as knowing your craft. You will succeed if you show that you can help editors to produce a successful publication. Once you accept this principle, only a little thought is needed. Keep your lines of communication open; at least get a telephone answering machine or set up a system by which editors can contact you. Jobs go to the easily available, and many people lose out because they cannot be traced.

Consider what support you will need. Make stationery and business cards an early priority. Beware making them too flashy, and avoid making claims that you cannot sustain. Putting 'writer and script consultant' on your card may look good, but it will be counterproductive if you do not have the expertise. A good wordprocessing package will help you with your administration, such as invoicing, book-keeping and letter writing. But such gadgets are intended to make your life easier, and not become an end in themselves.

You may also find it useful to invest in a filing cabinet, probably second-hand. Use it for storing your notes and records in case of any comebacks, and for keeping ideas and background information which you can dig out, flesh out and send out. This will be particularly useful if you decide to specialize in a particular area.

However – and I do not apologize for raising this point yet again – sophisticated systems are no use if you fail to deliver the goods. The essence of professionalism lies not in smart stationery or sophisticated software but in a conscientious and ethical approach. If you have that, you should have no problems.

Other types of writing

Do not feel ashamed if you decide not to branch out into other areas. Other types of writing involve different skills. Writers tend to be better at some than they are at others, and, more important still, are better at these than other writers. The trick is to know what you are good at, stick to it, and stop eyeing jealously the achievements of others.

With this warning in mind, I should stress that, should you choose to branch out, many of the principles discussed in this book will stand you in good stead. In particular you should understand the all-important attitude, which is that the needs of the audience are paramount. This is the key to successful communication. Also, you will have realized the importance of planning: the five stages – setting the brief, research, planning, writing and rewriting again – applies to most communication. But there are some differences, and the following sections are intended to show some of them. However, it only claims to be an appetizer, and to succeed in many of these fields you will need to invest in another book.

News stories

Our familiarity with news stories masks the fact that good ones are hard to write. They are relatively short, and each one has to compete for attention with many others. They call for careful analysis, good presentation, and concise, accurate writing.

The key is the first paragraph, which must tell the story and grab attention at the same time. From there the job is relatively simple: the accepted structure is known as the inverted pyramid, where points are fleshed out in order of importance. This has an important technical reason: news stories often have to be cut at the last minute, and it makes this process much easier if they can be cut from the bottom.

The market for news stories, however, is difficult. Most publications have their own news writers, and rarely take items from outside contributors. Payment usually depends on the number of lines published, and, because news stories are usually short, will tend to be poor. However, the technique is particularly useful for developing brevity, and you may sometimes be called upon to use it, for example if an editor asks you to cover a conference. Harold Evans explains it well in *Newsman's English*[29].

The technique can be adapted to press releases, which are essentially news stories written for a promotional purpose. The same principles apply, but you should make sure that you send it out on the organization's official notepaper, clearly dated and marked PRESS RELEASE, and with a heading, summarizing the main point. Make sure you put one or two contact numbers at the end of the release and that someone is available at them at the time when reporters are likely to ring.

Science writing

Scientific papers play an important part in the life of any doctor, and the new discipline of 'journalology' is growing up around them, dealing with matters such as refereeing systems, fraud, freedom to publish, and the role of journals. Some commentators have pointed out that this type of writing has purposes other than simple communication. For instance, Michael Shortland and Jane Gregory argue: 'Scientific publications have purposes other than the communication of ideas: they represent the productivity and therefore the 'value' of the research team; they establish hierarchies by the ordering of their author lines and by whom they choose to cite; and, most importantly of all, they serve the needs of their authors above the needs of their readers.'[30]

Nevertheless original papers remain for doctors a useful way of advancing knowledge and career. They may seem far removed from feature articles, but many of the techniques would be relevant. In particular, the first stage – setting the brief – will ensure that you have a clear idea of your hypothesis and your potential outlet before you start. The final stage – revision – will help you ask the right questions before you submit your paper.

But there are three important differences. First, because the main goal of publication is, to use Robert Day's[31] phrase, 'shine a spotlight on one area of the truth', your research will have to be more rigorous. Second, there is a widely accepted formula, the IMRAD structure, which should make the planning easier. This structure consists of Introduction (why we did it?), Method (what we did), Results (what we found) And Discussion (what it means). Third, you may need to adopt a more formal style when writing. The first audience you will have to satisfy will be the referees, and you should adopt a tone with which they will be comfortable, even though this may mean breaking some of our guidelines about short words and active voice. Most scientific publications now have Notes For Authors, and you should study these carefully before you start to write.

Not all scientific writing consists of original papers, and you should be aware of other possibilities, such as conference reports, review articles and editorials. Useful advice is contained in Robert Day's book *How To Write and Publish a Scientific Paper*[31], and in *Writing Successfully in Science* by Maeve O'Connor[32].

Novels

Most people feel they have a novel in them; few find out. The lessons of this book, such as the need for hard work and an effective style, once learnt, will stand you in good stead. But there are several important differences.

The most fundamental concerns the writer's basic approach. Throughout this book I have stressed the importance of writing for the reader, on the grounds that the main point of written communication is to get across information and ideas in the best possible way. Novelists, on the other hand, can write primarily for themselves in the sense that they invent a fictional creation whose primary purpose is to satisfy them. If this creation is good, it will be read and enjoyed; if not, it will not be published. It is a game played for far higher stakes and rewards for writer and reader are correspondingly higher.

There are also some technical differences. The scale of a novel, at between 30,000 and 60,000 words, is far greater and the discipline needed is correspondingly fiercer: at an average of 350 words a day, one draft could take three to six months. Quotation marks serve a different function: in journalism they are used to signal opinions which enliven and enlarge the argument, but in novels they are an essential part of the action. If they fail to advance the narrative, as in the *Hello, how are you?/ Very well thank-you* variety, they are useless.

Many people have written about writing novels, and for obvious reasons I would commend those by practising writers rather than by critics. A useful place to start is John Braine's *Writing a Novel* (Methuen, 1974)[33], which is accessible and sensible.

Broadcasting

It is easy to watch the presenters on *Tomorrow's World* or *Breakfast Television* and say: *I can do that*. But it is not just a question of turning up and talking. The usual journalistic qualities will be of help, particularly the ability to plan and to pitch your material at a level which attracts and keeps your audience. However, you will also need the indefinable quality of looking or sounding not just plausible, but authoritative, which many people simply cannot do. It may be purely a question of physiology, such as a high voice, slight lisp, or apparently shifty manner. If you can't do it, cut your losses at an early stage and go back to writing.

If you still think you can, how do you break in? The usual rules apply: get yourself known, possibly by building up a reputation as an expert in a particular area, or by starting in the relatively calmer atmosphere of a local radio station. Then build on your contacts. If you write frequently you will find that some day someone in the broadcast media will want to follow up your story, perhaps with an interview. Make the most of this contact.

Rewards are more likely to come from the buzz of performing rather than from a flurry of cheques, which will probably be of lower value than you might expect, and, in the case of local radio, non-existent. However, if you become really established, you will find yourself being approached for video presentations or for 'voice-overs', where you could get paid in the region of £1,000 a performance.

Video

Many independent producers put out videos, a lot of them sponsored by pharmaceutical companies. These range from the promotional to the educational, and they all have to be written. Again, your approach as a journalist will come in useful, but there will also be important differences, notably the ability to think in terms of images as well as words.

Target suitable producers by looking in the pharmaceutical industry reference book *Pharmafile*. Then write round with ideas. Producers will need to be satisfied that you can deliver what you have promised. If they like the idea, they will try to sell it to a sponsor. If successful, they will ask you to write the treatment, and pay you about £200. If the treatment is accepted, and you are asked to write the script, you should stand to earn about £1,000 a programme.

Writing plays

These seem a world away from writing articles, but many people, such as Tom Stoppard, have bridged the gap. Writers in this medium say that their priorities are plotting and structure, and getting involved with their characters. If they get this right, they will attract their audience. With most plays there is also a visual element to be considered.

However, one of the best places to start, the radio, lacks this characteristic. The BBC produce a useful eight-page leaflet for those interested in this market. 'Since it is a medium of almost unlimited possibilities, it calls for great discipline of structure and awareness of the nuances of language on the part of the writer,' it says. It gives advice on some of the major technical problems (like establishing who is speaking) and gives an example of laying out a script. It also contains a useful list of further reading plus addresses and markets within BBC Radio[34]. But be warned: the corporation receives about 200 scripts a week and may be considering more than 1,000 at any one time.

Pharmaceutical companies

Some of the highest rewards for the skilled medical writer come from the pharmaceutical industry, which each year puts out hundreds of product-related documents, such as patient-information leaflets, conference proceedings, conference newsletters, abstracts, and press information packs. You will need a good understanding of medical science, the ability to put complex ideas across simply, and, inevitably, reliability. Payment is usually higher than for independent publications, currently between £200 and £400 a day, and there can be the added bonus of paid-for foreign travel.

Some writers feel that accepting payment from the industry is wrong because it could be seen to compromise their independence. My own view is that, in a world of expanding information, there is nothing wrong in being paid for putting forward a point of view. However, writers should never put their name to an article if they do not feel comfortable with it, and should always make it clear if they have a vested financial interest. Some public relations companies have paid journalists to write about their products and then submit this article, without mentioning this prior commission, to an independent publication. This is clearly dishonest, and the Medical Journalists Association has rightly condemned it.

This market is highly competitive, and those who wish to break into it should make sure that they have had sufficient experience. Write to public relations consultancies and to the public relations departments of pharmaceutical industries with a CV and samples of your work.

Desktop publishing

If you cannot find anyone to publish your work, the arrival of relatively cheap desktop publishing systems now means that you can publish it yourself. You will need to own, or have access to, a desktop publishing system. This will comprise a hardware system (personal computer, keyboard and screen) and, preferably, a laser printer. You will also need the right software: a word processing package, and a desktop publishing package, such as Ventura or Pagemaker at the top of the scale, or one of the less expensive ones such as Timeworks or Fleet Street Editor. This will enable you to write and edit your articles and arrange them electronically on the page. When you get more ambitious, you will be able to add a graphics package, which will enable you to illustrate your publication. A good system will cost upwards of £3,000. You can print the finished work on your laser printer and a photocopier, or send it to a professional printing house.

You must decide who is to be the editor, and therefore responsible for the publication. This is a legal requirement, but it is also good practice because it will set out clear lines of responsibility from the start. As the editor, you will have to balance getting the publication read, with steering clear of major political difficulties, and making money.

Set out a statement of intent. What is the publication for? How will

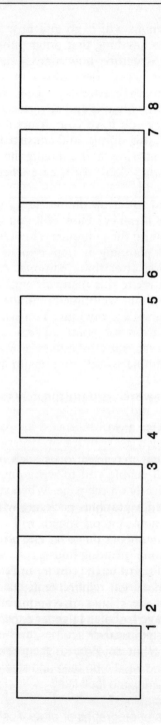

Figure 10.1 Flatplan

Publication:

Edition:

you produce it? To whom will it go and how will it get there? Who will write it? Will it do anything that other publications don't or can't do? Work out a clear structure: how many pages you will need – and can afford – and then write them down in a flat plan (see Figure 10.1). Then allocate to each page the items, such as news, features, readers' letters, editorial, columns and advertisements, that you propose running regularly. Once you have your structure, decide on the design (see Figure 10.2). Keep this simple, and consistent: whenever magazines have experimented by moving their contents the readers have sent back the clear message that they don't really care where things go, but please stop moving them around.

Finally you will need to set up the necessary systems. How will you fill the news pages, for instance? How will you get the advertisements? Who, if anyone, will write the columns? These have to be done edition after edition, so early planning is important if you are to avoid the common fate of folding after three editions. Arthur Plotnik suggests that all editors should recite this mantra: 'Nothing happens when it is supposed to happen without well-timed reminders'[35].

The rewards, of course, are obvious. You will have the opportunity to write, to put forward your point of view and to carry the views of others. You may even start to influence events. If you are really successful you will be able to sell to a major publisher and retire to the South of France.

Such an outcome, however, is unfortunately rare.

Figure 10.2 Design house style

These are some of the questions to ask when drawing up a design house style:

1. What should be the size, weight and colour of the paper?
2. How many pages should the publication be?
3. How many columns should there be and what should be the width of the columns?
4. What type face and size should I use for body text?
5. Should text be set right, left, centred or justified?
6. What type face and size should I use for the headlines?
7. What type face and size should I use for captions?
8. How should I use white space?
9. How should I use other devices, such as standfirsts, quotes, cross-heads, dingbats, and what type face and size should they be?
10. What should the nameplate look like?
11. Will I be able to use colour?
12. Will I be able to use photographs or other illustration?

Training and careers

Further training

More and more people are starting to write, which means that more and more people are writing books for them. Go to any bookshop and you will see a large array, ranging from writing for specialist markets to personal reminiscences to sociological critiques of the mass media. Appendix 1 contains a mainly personal list, plus a general reading list given to postgraduate students at City University, London. You should be aware that reading is seductive, and that there comes a point where writing should take its place.

But writing can be a lonely business, and those who practise it often feel the need for what Michael O'Donnell calls 'patient support groups'. That is, writers who meet regularly to share their problems with like-minded others. There are writers' circles throughout the country, and many local authorities run evening classes. Check these out carefully: if they are biased towards romantic fiction they may not be what you need.

There are also a number of professional organizations, such as the Medical Journalists Association or the British Science Writers Association which organize regular meetings, sponsor competitions and usually provide some sort of newsletter. A list is attached to Appendix 2. The most important function is that they provide links with writers and editors.

For those who want more formal training, the past few years has seen a large rise in the number of courses run by colleges, polytechnics and universities, and in the private sector. These include six-month or one-year postgraduate courses and also various short courses. Some private organizations provide correspondence courses: the problem with these is that it is difficult to keep motivated. There is a list of some of the main providers in Appendix 3. Standards vary, and, as a rough guide, you should check whether they have been approved by accreditation groups like the National Council for the Training of Journalists (for newspapers) and the Periodicals Training Council (for magazines).

Full-time careers

Over the past few years I have met a steady stream of doctors who wish to leave medicine for journalism. My first piece of advice is know what's involved. As Lowry and Smith write: 'Journalists ...rank no better than politicians or union leaders and are thought of as mendacious, unfeeling, greedy or drunken...This sudden drop in status may put some aspiring doctors off while it may positively attract others.' If this does not this does not deter you, try to find out more about the jobs that attract you, and decide which particular aspects – such as reporting, specialist writing, sub-editing, editing, broadcasting – that you would be happy doing. Beware dropping off one treadmill onto another.

Don't expect to get your ideal job immediately because you will almost certainly need some training. A medical degree can be useful in journalism, particularly if you will be writing about medicine, but it is not enough. There are other specific skills you need to master before you can be a valuable member of an editorial team.

There are two ways of getting that training. The first is to get onto one of the reputable postgraduate courses. Until recently, graduates from these schemes were almost guaranteed a job at the end of their course, but the recession has meant that many graduating in 1991 have found it hard to get places; this is expected to last for at least another year. Therefore the second avenue is probably more fruitful at the moment: this involves getting a job with a major publisher who will undertake to provide the training you need.

Goodbye – and good luck

Our journey is now complete, though I hope that yours is just beginning. It remains for me to wish you every success in writing. I hope that you will get as much pleasure out of it as I have done.

Alex Paton quotes a journalist friend who, when asked how he managed to write with such ease, replied 'The first million words are the worst'. Michael O'Donnell has pointed out that 'The greater the suffering while the stuff is being hammered out the greater the joy when you reach the last full stop.'[36]

Quite, and here it is –.

Key points

1. If you wish to continue writing, develop your contacts. Aim at being in the position of being commissioned. This requires a professional approach.
2. If you wish to move out into one of the many related fields, many of the guidelines in this book will be useful. But there are important differences.
3. If you want further training, many courses and 'support groups' are available.
4. If you want to become a full-time journalist, you will need further training.

References

(1) Paton A (1985) Write a Paper. In *How to Do It 1*, 2nd edition, p207. BMJ Books.

(2) Gowers Sir E (1986) *The Complete Plain Words*, 3rd edition, revised by Greenbaum S and Whitcut J, p39. Her Majesty's Stationery Office.

(3) Hennessy B (1989) *Writing Feature Articles*, p245. Heinemann Professional Publishing.

(4) Braine J (1990) *Writing a Novel*, 3rd edition, p30. Methuen.

(5) Shortland M and Gregory J (1991) *Communicating Science, A Handbook*, p35. Longman Scientific and Technical.

(6) Op. cit. Hennessy, pxi.

(7) Periodical Publishers' Association, *Magazine Handbook 1991*.

(8) O'Donnell M (1987) Write for Money. In *How To Do It 2*, p197. BMJ Books.

(9) National Union of Journalists. *Who Owns What, 1988*.

(10) Day RE (1988) *How to Write and Publish a Scientific Paper*, 3rd edition, p94. Cambridge University Press.

(11) Plotnik A. (1982) *Elements of Editing*, p25. Collier Macmillan.

(12) Op. cit. Day, pix.

(13) Op. cit. Hennessy, p56.

(14) Durant JR, Evans GA, Thomas GP (1989) The Public Understanding of Science. In *Nature*, 340, pp11–14.

(15) Sellers L (1985) *The Simple Subs Book*, p64, 2nd edition. Pergamon Press.

(16) Whale J (1984) *Put It In Writing*, p14. JM Dent & Sons.

(17) Adams S (1985) A Guide to Editorial Practice. In *Periodical Journalism* pp42–44. Periodicals Training Council.

(18) Bottomley T, Loftus A (1971) *A Journalist's Guide to the Use of English*, p5. Express and Star Newspapers.

(19) Strunk Jr W, White EB (1979) *The Elements of Style*, 3rd edition, p66-70. Collier Macmillan.

(20) Evans H (1972) *Newsman's English*, pp20–33. Heinemann Professional Publishing.

(21) Op. cit. Gowers, p4.

(22) Albert T, Chadwick S (1991) *How Readable are Practice Leaflets, ????*.

(23) Op. cit. O'Donnell, p198.

(24) The New York Times (1976) *Manual of Style And Usage*, foreword. The New York Times Company.

(25) Op. cit. Gowers, p98.

(26) Brewis A (1990) Please an Editor. In *How To Do It 3*, p64. BMJ Books.

(27) Lowry S, Smith R (1985) Become A Medical Journalist or Editor. In *How To Do It 1*, p135. BMJ Books.

(28) Op. cit. O'Donnell, p199.

(29) Op. cit. Evans.

(30) Op. cit. Shortland, p51.

(31) Op. cit. Day, p45.

(32) O'Connor M (1991) *Writing Successfully in Science*. Harper Collins Academic.

(33) Braine J (1974) *Writing a Novel*. Methuen.

(34) *Writing Plays for Radio*, available from BBC Radio.

(35) Op. cit. Plotnik, p6.

(36) Op. cit. Paton, p211.

Appendix 1: Selected Reading

Journalism techniques

GETTING THE WORDS RIGHT, Theodore Cheney, Writers Digest, 1983: only book which describes the mechanics and importance of editing, rewriting and revising material.

NEWSMAN'S ENGLISH, Harold Evans, Heinemann Professional Publishing Ltd, 1990: standard textbook for journalists. Excellent advice on use of English plus copious examples from news writing.

WRITING FEATURE ARTICLES, Brendan Hennessy, Heinemann Professional Publishing Ltd, 1989: thorough look at writing and marketing.

THE SIMPLE SUBS BOOK, Leslie Sellers, Pergamon Press, 1985: another journalists' classic. Slightly dated but fun, and useful insight into the way sub-editors work.

Effective writing

A JOURNALIST'S GUIDE TO THE USE OF ENGLISH, Ted Bottomley and Anthony Loftus, Express and Star Newspapers, 1980: excellent sections on syntax and punctuation for those who want remedial education without too many long words.

THE ELEMENTS OF STYLE, William Strunk Jr and E B White, Macmillan Publishing Co Inc, 3rd edition, 1979: blessedly slim classic, with rules of usage, principles of composition, matters of form, commonly misused words and expressions and 21 reminders on good style.

EFFECTIVE WRITING, Christopher Tuck and John Kirkman, Span, 1989: comprehensive coverage of scientific, technical and business communication.

PUT IT IN WRITING, John Whale, Dent Paperbacks, 1984: elegant series of essays, first published in the *Sunday Times*, on some of the main issues of style. Sample chapters: *Punctuation as Timing, The Little-Used Hyphen* and *Sparing the Reader Pain*. Quotes wide range of contemporary writers, from Anita Brookner to Helen McInnes.

THE COMPLETE PLAIN WORDS, Sir Ernest Gowers, 3rd edition revised by Sidney Greenbaum and Janet Whitcut, HMSO, 1986: civil servant's classic advice on 'the intricacies of the English language'. Useful to quote as final arbiter.

Specialized writing

WRITING SUCCESSFULLY IN SCIENCE, Maeve O'Connor, Harper Collins Academic, 1991: latest work from secretary-treasurer of the European Association of Science Editors. Thorough review of the subject.

HOW TO WRITE AND PUBLISH A SCIENTIFIC PAPER, Robert A Day (3rd edition), Cambridge University Press, 3rd edition 1989: hilarious and informative. Good after-dinner stories for scientific gatherings.

COMMUNICATING SCIENCE, A HANDBOOK, Michael Shortland and Jane Gregory, Longman Scientific and Technical, 1991: entertaining and persuasive argument on the need for scientists to communicate, with practical sections on writing, speaking and 'meeting the media'. Peppered with epigrams.

THORNE'S BETTER MEDICAL WRITING, Stephen Lock, Pitman Medical, 1977: authoritative 'primer on medical authorship' revised by the former editor of the *BMJ*.

WRITING A NOVEL, John Braine, 3rd edition 1990, Methuen: highly readable advice for intending novelists.

Editing

THE ELEMENTS OF EDITING, Arthur Plotnik, Collier Macmillan, 1982: companion to Strunk and White. Some useful advice on editing.

Miscellaneous

BMJ HOW-TO-DO-IT, 1- 3, BMJ Books, 1985, 1987, 1990: useful series with concise advice on a broad range of topics. Those relevant to writers include *Become a Medical Journalist or Editor, Be Your Own Subeditor, Deal with a Publisher (vol I), Write for Money, Choose a Better Word (vol II), Choose a Word Processor, Please an Editor (vol III)*.

MCNAE'S ESSENTIAL LAW FOR JOURNALISTS, Tom Welsh and Walter Greenwood, Vol II, 1990. Butterworths: useful handbook for the nervous. Constantly revised and updated.

PERIODICAL JOURNALISM: A GUIDE TO EDITORIAL PRACTICE, Periodicals Training Council (under revision): broad sweep of magazines, including writing, copy preparation, layout and design, law and production.

DOCTORING THE MEDIA, Anne Karpf, Routledge, 1988: challenging analysis of the coverage of health and medical issues in the media.

Freelancing

SUCCESSFUL FREELANCE JOURNALISM, Fay Goldie, OUP 1984: introduction to problems of writing and marketing freelance work.

BUSINESS OF FREELANCING, Graham Jones, BFP 1991: covers financial aspects of freelancing.

Reference books

WRITERS' AND ARTISTS' YEARBOOK, A & C Black, published annually: long-established guide with information on markets etc, plus useful articles on subjects of interest, such as libel and copyright.

THE WRITERS' HANDBOOK, Macmillan Reference, published annually: relatively new competitor to above with some differences of emphasis and presentation.

PHARMAFILE: standard reference work on pharmaceutical industry, with sections on publications, video producers. Also has section on publishing. Published by Pharmafile, Tower House, Southampton Street, London WC2E 7LS.

ECONOMIST STYLE BOOK: originating in-house at the *Economist*. Now widely adopted by 'heavy' institutions as their guide book.

OXFORD WRITERS DICTIONARY, OUP, 1990: desk companion for all writers offering direction on usage and definitions of most-used words.

OXFORD DICTIONARY FOR SCIENTIFIC WRITERS AND EDITORS, OUP, 1991: as above, but concentrating on scientific and medical subjects.

This booklist was compiled with the help of David Simmonds of L. Simmonds, specialists in journalism books, 16 Fleet Street, London EC4Y 1AX (071 353 3907).

General reading

These are books recommended to postgraduate students of journalism at City University, London.

THE BBC – THE FIRST FIFTY YEARS, Asa Briggs, OUP.
FOURTH-RATE ESTATE, AN ANATOMY OF FLEET STREET, Tom Baistow, Comedia, 1985.
POINT OF DEPARTURE, James Cameron, Granada Publishing, 1980.
DOG EAT DOG: CONFESSIONS OF A TABLOID JOURNALIST, Wensley Clarkson, Fourth Estate, 1990.
THE MAKING OF THE INDEPENDENT, Michael Clozier, Gordon Fraser Gallery, 1988.
POWER WITHOUT RESPONSIBILITY, James Curran and Jean Seaton, Routledge.
THE MADWOMAN'S UNDERCLOTHES, Germaine Greer, Picador, 1986–7.
BY-LINE, Ernest Hemingway, Penguin, 1980.
MODERN NEWSPAPER PRACTICE, F W Hodgson, Heinemann.
DISPATCHES, Michael Herr, Picador, 1977.
NEWS, NEWSPAPERS AND TELEVISION, Alastair Hetherington, Macmillan, 1985.
THE FIRST CASUALTY, Phillip Knightley, Quartet Books, 1980.
EDDY SHAH: TODAY AND THE NEWSPAPER REVOLUTION, Brian MacArthur, David and Charles 1988.

THE COLLECTED ESSAYS, JOURNALISM AND LETTERS, George Orwell, Penguin, 1971.
HEROES, John Pilger, Cape, 1986.
THE LITERARY JOURNALISTS, Norman Sims, Ballantine, New York, 1984.

Appendix 2: Useful names and addresses

Professional organizations

ASSOCIATION OF BRITISH SCIENCE WRITERS, c/ o Sue Lowell, the British Association for the Advancement of Science, Fortress House, 23 Savile Row, London W1X 1AB (Tel: 071 494 3326): about 350 members in radio, TV and print media plus relevant press and PR officers. Organizes visits and meetings, administers annual award, publishes monthly newsletter. Doctors usually eligible as associates. Cost: £15 full; £12 associate.

ASSOCIATION OF BROADCASTING DOCTORS, Peter Petts, Director, PO Box 15, Ely, Cambridge CB7 4SG (Tel: 0353 88456): about 300 members. Organizes training meetings, coordinates campaigns and provides liaison service. Cost: £25 pa.

COMEDY WRITERS ASSOCIATION OF GREAT BRITAIN, Ken Rock, Chairman, Ashmore Park, Wolverhampton, W Midlands WV11 2PS (Tel: 0902 722729): about 75 members. Local meetings, annual seminar in London and writers' weekend. Quarterly magazine with market information. Doctors eligible on published work or through entrance test. Cost: £30 pa plus £5 entrance fee.

GP WRITERS ASSOCIATION, Jill Byrne, the Cottage, 102A High Street, Henley in Arden, Solihull, West Midlands B95 5BY, Tel: 0564 794894): about 250 members. Newsletter, directory, award and two conferences a year. GP writers are eligible and non-GPs writing about general practice. Cost: £15 pa.

INSTITUTE OF JOURNALISTS, Bill Tadd, 2 Dock Offices, Surrey Quays, London SE16 2XL (Tel: 071 252 1187): professional body and independent (non- TUC) trade union. About 2,000 members. Protects members in exercise of professional duties and in their employment. Doctors eligible as affiliates. Cost: £75pa (affiliates).

MEDICAL JOURNALISTS ASSOCIATION, 14 Hovendens, Sissing-hurst, Cranbrook, Kent TN17 2LA (Tel: 0580 713920): about 300 members who write and broadcast about medicine and health. Doctors normally eligible as affiliates. Runs meetings, organizes awards and acts as professional pressure group. Cost: £20 pa.

NATIONAL UNION OF JOURNALISTS, Acorn House, 314 Gray's Inn Road, London WC1X 8DP (Tel: (071 278 7916): TUC-affiliated union 25,000 members in Britain and Republic of Ireland. Concerned with terms and conditions, health and safety and professional matters, including freedom of expression. Members must earn majority of income from journalism. Cost: £48–165.

P.E.N., 7 Dilke Street, London SW3 4JE (Tel: 071 352 6303): about 1,000 Members. English centre for International P.E.N. International congresses, regular Wednesday literary lectures, annual open day. Fights for freedom to write. Doctors who have published full length book by reputable publisher are eligible. Cost: £25 (London), £20 (country).

THE PENMAN CLUB, Leonard G Stubbs, General Secretary, 175 Pall Mall, Leigh-on-Sea, Essex SS9 1RE (Tel: 0702 74438): about 4,000 members internationally. Free criticism and advice plus use of postal library. Doctors (published or unpublished) eligible. Cost: £8.25 pa plus £3 entry fee.

THE SOCIETY OF AUTHORS (Medical Writers' Group), 84 Drayton Gardens, London SW10 9SB (Tel: 071 373 6642): 5,000 members, with about 220 members, mainly medically qualified, in the group. Independent trade union which provides advisory service, organizes lectures and seminars, administers annual award. Cost: £65 pa (£47 for under 35s).

SOCIETY OF WOMEN WRITERS AND JOURNALISTS, Jean Hawkes, Secretary, 110 Whitehall Road, Chingford, London E4 6DW: free advice for members and monthly lunchtime meetings and work-shops in London. *The Woman Journalist* three times a year. Women doctors who have published are eligible. Cost: £18 pa (town); £15 pa (country).

WOMEN WRITERS NETWORKS, Susan Kerr, Vice-chair, 55 Burlington Lane, LONDON W4 3ET (Tel: 081 994 1598): about 150 members. Provides forum for information, support and networking. Monthly meetings in London. Women doctors eligible (published or unpublished). Cost: £20 pa.

WRITING CIRCLES, Jill Dick, Horderns Park Road, Chapel-en-le-Frith, Derbyshire SK12 6SY: will send directory of writers' circles for £3.

Training organizations

Full-time training

CENTRE FOR JOURNALISM STUDIES, University of Wales, College of Cardiff (UWCC), 69 Park Place, Cardiff, CF1 3AA. (Tel: 0222 874786): one year postgraduate diploma course with options in newspaper, magazine or broadcast media. 60 places (1,000 applicants). Cost: £2,630 tuition fees (1991–2), applications close February 15.

CITY UNIVERSITY, Northampton Square, London EC1V 0HB (Tel: 071 253 4399): one year full-time postgraduate diploma in international/ newspaper/ periodical/ broadcast journalism. About 700 applicants for 100 palaces. Cost: £2,600 (1991–2). Also short courses, including freelance writing and sub-editing.

IMPERIAL COLLEGE, (Ros Herman), Sherfield Building, London SW7 2AE (Tel: 071 589 5111 X 7060): one year full-time or two year part-time MSc in science communication (media, museums, communications theory) started in 1991. 13 students (30 applicants). Cost: £2,100.

LANCASHIRE POLYTECHNIC, Centre for Journalism, Music Centre, Edward Street, Preston, PR1 2TQ (Tel: 0772 201201 ext 2501): postgraduate diploma in newspaper (40 places) or radio and TV journalism (25 places). Applications: Nov-Jan. Cost: £716 (1991–2).

LONDON COLLEGE OF PRINTING, Elephant and Castle, London SE1 6SB. (Tel: 071 735 9100 ext 2611): 13 week postgraduate course in periodical journalism, starting in January and September. Cost: £208. Also evening courses.

GLASGOW POLYTECHNIC, Cowcaddens Road, Glasgow G4 0BA (Tel: 041 331 3268): one year postgraduate diploma in journalism (jointly with Strathclyde University). 20 students (200 applicants). Cost: £3,000 (1991–92).

REED BUSINESS PUBLISHING GROUP, Fabian Acker, Quadrant House, The Quadrant, Sutton, Surrey, SM2 5AS. (Tel: 081 661 3956): 17 week full-time course in magazine journalism, starting January and August. Cost: £2,232. Also correspondence course, including two days' face-to-face tuition and six months' NUJ membership on application). Cost: £500. Also short courses.

Part-time training

POLYTECHNIC OF CENTRAL LONDON, School of Communications, 18–22 Riding House Street, London W1P 7PD (Tel: 071 911 5000): Part-time MA (Two to three years). Cost: £140–160 for each module. Short courses only.

PMA TRAINING, The Old Anchor, Church Street, Hemingford Grey, Cambs PE18 9DF (Tel: 0480 300653): nine-week introductory course from July to September. Postgraduate. 24 places. 1991 cost: £1,500. Applications close in April. Also short courses for professional journalists.

TIM ALBERT & ASSOCIATES, 5 Cobham Road, Leatherhead, Surrey KT22 9AU. (Tel: 0372 377848): short courses (open and in-house) on medical journalism, setting up publications, science writing etc. Advisory service.

WRITE HANDS, Tea Warehouse, 10A Lant Street, London SE1 1QR: two day introduction to journalism in September. Covers opportunities and techniques for finding a job. Cost: £225 (1991).

Many colleges and polytechnics now run courses in journalism. The following are listed as accredited by the National Council for the Training of Journalists:

Cardiff Institute of Higher Education (0222 551111)
Darlington College of Technology (0325 467651)
Harlow College (0279 441288)
Highbury College, Portsmouth (0705 383131)
Stradbroke College, Sheffield (0742 392621)
Lancashire Polytechnic (see above)
Napier Polytechnic of Edinburgh (031 444 2266)
The Belfast Institute of Further and Higher Education (0232 245891)
City University, London (see above)
University of Wales College of Cardiff (see above)
North East Wales Institute, Wrexham (0978 290666)
Calderdale College, Halifax (0422 358221)
West Surrey College of Art and Design, Farnham (0252 722441)
Cornwall College of Further Education, Redruth (0209 712911)

Miscellaneous

NATIONAL COUNCIL FOR THE TRAINING OF JOURNALISTS, Carlton House, Hemnall Street, Epping, Essex, CM16 4NL (Tel: 0378 72395): administers national certificate in newspaper journalism and runs short courses. Can provide list of colleges and universities providing full-time courses in journalism.

PERIODICALS TRAINING COUNCIL, Imperial House, 15–19 Kings-way, London WC2B 6UN (Tel: 071 836 8798): runs courses (including three week block release) and overseas training for magazine journalists. Advises on training.

BRITISH MEDICAL JOURNAL, BMA House Tavistock Square, London WC1H 9JR (tel: 071 387 4499): one year registrarship for doctors three to five years after qualifying. Salary £25,500 (1991–2). Apply in Autumn to start in March. Also annual Clegg Scholarship: an eight week attachment for medical students. Apply in Autumn for following year.

BMA NEWS REVIEW, BMA House, Tavistock Square, London WC1H 9JR (tel: 071 387 4499): one day introductory courses on medical journalism. 1992 cost: £75 + VAT (BMA members).

Appendix 3: NUJ Code of Professional Conduct

1. A journalist has a duty to maintain the highest professional and ethical standards.

2. A journalist shall at all times defend the principle of the freedom of the press and other media in relation to the collection of information and the expression of comment and criticism. He/she shall strive to eliminate distortion, news suppression and censorship.

3. A journalist shall strive to ensure that the information he/she disseminates is fair and accurate, avoid the expression of comment and conjecture as established fact and falsification by distortion, selection or misrepresentation.

4. A journalist shall rectify promptly any harmful inaccuracies, ensure that correction and apologies receive due prominence and afford the right of reply to persons criticized when the issue is of sufficient importance.

5. A journalist shall obtain information, photographs and illustrations only by straightforward means. The use of other means can be justified only by overriding consideration of the public interest. The journalist is entitled to exercise a personal conscientious objection to the use of such means.

6. Subject to justification by overriding considerations of the public interest, a journalist shall do nothing which entails intrusion into private grief and distress.

7. A journalist shall protect confidential sources of information.

8. A journalist shall not accept bribes nor shall he/she allow other inducements to influence the performance of his/her professional duties.

9. A journalist shall not lend himself/herself to the distortion or suppression of the truth because of advertising or other considerations.

10. A journalist shall only mention a person's race, colour, creed, illegitimacy, marital status or lack of it, gender or sexual orientation if this information is strictly relevant. A journalist shall neither originate nor process material which encourages discrimination on any of the above-mentioned grounds.

11. A journalist shall not take private advantage of information gained in the course of his/her duties, before the information is public knowledge.

12. A journalist shall not by way of statement, voice or appearance endorse by advertisement any commercial product or service save for the promotion of his/her own work or of the medium by which he/she is employed.

Appendix 4: Useful terms

ADVERTISING: paid-for material advocating goods or services. Finances writers, whether they like it or not. Can be **display** or **classified**.

ADVERTORIAL: articles which advertisers have paid for. Should not be allowed to masquerade as independent editorial matter.

ANGLE: way of approaching each feature or news story. Preferably different from (but not worse than) angle chosen by anyone else.

BODY COPY: type style of main text, as distinct from **display type**, which is the style or styles chosen for headlines, captions etc.

BRIEF: (1) clear statement of intent for each article; (2) one paragraph news story, also called **Nib** (News In Brief).

BY-LINE: author's name displayed prominently on an article.

CATCHLINE: short identifying label on the top of each page of copy.

CAPTION: words explaining a picture, drawing or diagram. Usually written by sub-editors.

CLIPPINGS: items that have already appeared in print on a person or event. Also **cuttings**.

CONTACT: journalist's name for someone who will be useful to him. Not to be confused with **friends**.

CONTROLLED CIRCULATION: practice of sending publications to a target readership, whether they want it or not.

COPY: a noun which refers to written words destined for a publication.

COPY FIT: to make an article fit the space available. Sometimes painful.

COVER STORY: article in a magazine which is featured on the front cover.

CROSSHEAD: a word or short phrase in display type which appears in the middle of a column of text. Mainly a visual device.

CONTACTS BOOK: index of useful names, addresses etc. Essential to successful freelancing.

CUTS: words removed from an article in order to make it fit allotted space. Disliked by authors, but often improves their work.

DEADLINE: not an abstract concept, but a date by which a certain task needs to be done if the publication is to be produced on time.
DESKTOP PUBLISHING: software which enables pages to be laid out electronically.

EDITOR: the person who is ultimately responsible for a publication.
EDITORIAL: (1) all articles, illustrations etc; distinct from advertising; (2) article reflecting opinion of the publication. Doesn't have to be pompous.

FEATURE: an article of 800–2,000 words, longer and sometimes more opinionated than a **news story**.
FLAT PLAN one-dimensional representation of all the pages of a publication. Essential tool for planning.
FREELANCE: a writer of variable standard who is not a paid staff member of the publication.

HACK: term for journalist. Now often considered a compliment, and superseded as term of abuse by **reptile**.
HANDOUT: a press release promoting a product, event etc.
HARD COPY: article written on paper (as opposed to disk).
HEADLINE: a means of enticing readers into an article with a short phrase or sentence in larger letters (**display type**).
HOUSE STYLE: rules on style laid down by the editor.

INTERVIEW: process of getting information face-to-face or over a telephone.
INTRO: the opening part of a story.

KILL FEE: payment for an article which has been commissioned but will not be used.

LAYOUT: plan showing position of text, headlines, pictures etc.
LEAD STORY: most prominent and most important news story in publication or on page (**page lead**).
LEAD TIME: period between writing an article and seeing it in print.
LIBEL: words held to lower someone's reputation and (if the court decides) can subsequently raise their capital.
LINEAGE: practice of paying writers according to the number of lines printed. Pronounced in two syllables.
LITERAL: a spelling mistake. American usage: **typo**.
LUNCH: well-tested technique for gathering information, cultivating contacts and producing ideas. Not liked by accountants.

OFF-DIARY: story that does not come from predictable event, like court appearance or meeting.

OFF THE RECORD: an agreement by writer and interviewee that the information about to be given cannot be used. **Non attributable** means that the information can be given, but without a source.

PAR or PARA: paragraph. With news stories, usually synonymous with sentences. Can be longer for features.
PEG: event used as excuse to give another outing to well-used facts.
PRESS CONFERENCE: a specially organized event, intended to be newsworthy, to which journalists are invited.
PRESS RELEASE: information put out by an organization in order to receive publicity.
PROOFREAD: An opportunity to change errors of fact and spelling mistakes; not a chance to revise opinions. Authors will be asked to do this on a **proof** or **galley (proof)**.
PUFF: an article which is so favourable to its subject that it looks like an advertisement.
PROFILE: word portrait of someone, compiled from a number of sources and not just one interview.
PUT TO BED: point at which an edition is sent to printers. Expensive to wake it up again after this point.

QUOTE: a quoted opinion from someone other than the author. Should be clearly labelled and used freely.

REFEREE: an expert called in to advise on a submitted article. In scientific publishing, this process is formalized (**peer review**).
RETAINER: sum of money paid to writer (usually annually) in return for specific duties (eg seven articles a year).

SCOOP: an exclusive story. Journalists use the term **exclusive**.
SPIKE: formerly a metal hook on a wooden base on which articles were stuck if unusable. Now used as a verb, to mean that a story has been shelved. This is different from a story being **killed**, which means that it must on no account be used.
STANDFIRST: a subsidiary headline, used as a second attempt to entice readers.
STRINGER: freelance journalist used by publication to report on a specific area. Often paid retainer.
SUBEDIT: the process of amending copy for style, readability, legality etc. Distinct from **editing**, which is the process of deciding whether the work is worth publishing in the first place.

UPPER CASE: capital letters, distinct from **lower case**.

WIDOW: single word at top of column. **Orphan** is single word at bottom of column. Considered ugly and generally eliminated.

Appendix 5: Proofmarks

Correcting proofs is one of those areas where a number of traditions has grown up.

The British standards Institution at Linford Wood, Milton Keynes, MK14 6LE has a list of the agreed marks in use in the UK. However, different marks are used in the USA and in Europe. The most important thing to do is make sure that your marks are legible. If they are, then a good subeditor or printer should be able to interpret them.

In double spaced manuscripts you should be able to make the marks in the text, where the typesetter will clearly see them.

WHEN you correcting a proof

WHEN you are correcting a proof make your mark clearly in the margin. Indicate in the text the exact spot where the change should be made.

Most important of all, remember that any proof reading you do will be useless if you do not meet the deadline.

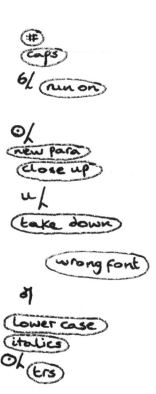

Correcting proofs is one of those areas where a number of traditions has grown up.

The British Standards Institution at Linford Wood, Milton Keynes, MK14 6LE has a list of the agreed marks in use in the UK. However, different marks are used in the USA and in Europe

The most important thing to do is make sure that your marks are legible. If they are, then a good sub-editor or printer should be able to interpret them.

In double spaced manuscripts you should be able to make the marks in the text, where the typesetter will clearly see them.

When you are correcting a proof make your mark *clearly* in the margin, Indicate in the text the exact spot where the change should be made.

Most important of all, remember that any proof reading you do will be useless if you do not meet the deadline.

Index